Exotic Animal Nutrition

Editor

AMANDA J. ARDENTE

VETERINARY CLINICS OF NORTH AMERICA: EXOTIC ANIMAL PRACTICE

www.vetexotic.theclinics.com

Consulting Editor
JÖRG MAYER

January 2024 • Volume 27 • Number 1

ELSEVIER

1600 John F. Kennedy Boulevard • Suite 1800 • Philadelphia, Pennsylvania, 19103-2899
http://www.vetexotic.theclinics.com

VETERINARY CLINICS OF NORTH AMERICA: EXOTIC ANIMAL PRACTICE Volume 27, Number 1
January 2024 ISSN 1094-9194, ISBN-13: 978-0-443-24632-6

Editor: Stacy Eastman
Developmental Editor: Varun Gopal

Veterinary Clinics of North America: Exotic Animal Practice (ISSN 1094-9194) is published in January, May, and September by Elsevier, Inc., 360 Park Avenue South, New York, NY 10010-1710. Subscription prices are $311.00 per year for US individuals, $100.00 per year for US students and residents, $362.00 per year for Canadian individuals, $377.00 per year for international individuals, $100.00 per year Canadian students/residents, and $165.00 per year for international students/residents. For institutional access pricing please contact Customer Service via the contact information below. To receive student/resident rate, orders must be accompanied by name of affiliated institution, date of term, and the *signature* of program/residency coordinator on institution letterhead. Orders will be billed at individual rate until proof of status is received. Foreign air speed delivery is included in all *Clinics* subscription prices. All prices are subject to change without notice. **POSTMASTER:** Send address changes to *Veterinary Clinics of North America: Exotic Animal Practice*, Elsevier Health Sciences Division, Subscription Customer Service, 3251 Riverport Lane, Maryland Heights, MO 63043. **Customer Service: Telephone: 1-800-654-2452** (U.S. and Canada); **1-314-447-8871** (outside U.S. and Canada). **Fax: 1-314-447-8029. E-mail: journalscustomerservice-usa@elsevier.com (for print support); journalsonlinesupport-usa@elsevier.com (for online support).**

Reprints. For copies of 100 or more of articles in this publication, please contact the Commercial Reprints Department, Elsevier Inc., 360 Park Avenue South, New York, New York 10010-1710. Tel.: 212-633-3874; Fax: 212-633-3820; E-mail: reprints@elsevier.com.

Veterinary Clinics of North America: Exotic Animal Practice is covered in *MEDLINE/PubMed (Index Medicus).*

Contributors

CONSULTING EDITOR

JÖRG MAYER, Dr med vet, MSc
Diplomate, American Board of Veterinary Practitioners (Exotic Companion Mammals);
Diplomate, European College of Zoological Medicine (Small Mammals); Diplomate,
American College of Zoological Medicine; Associate Professor of Zoological Medicine,
Department of Small Animal Medicine and Surgery, University of Georgia College of
Veterinary Medicine, Athens, Georgia, USA

EDITOR

AMANDA J. ARDENTE, DVM, PhD
Ardente Veterinary Nutrition, Ocala, Florida, USA

AUTHORS

TRINITA BARBOZA, DVM, DVSC
Department of Clinical Sciences, Zoological Companion Animal Medicine Service,
Cummings School of Veterinary Medicine at Tufts University, North Grafton,
Massachusetts, USA

MARJORIE BERCIER, DMV
Diplomate, American College of Zoological Medicine; Department of Clinical Sciences,
Zoological Companion Animal Medicine Service, Cummings School of Veterinary
Medicine at Tufts University, North Grafton, Massachusetts, USA

MATTHEW A. BROOKS, MS, PhD
Animalis Nutrition Consulting, LLC, Zionsville, Indiana, USA; NomNomNow, Inc, Nashville,
Tennessee, USA

**KARA M. BURNS, MS, MEd, LVT, VTS (Nutrition), VTS Hon (Internal Medicine,
Dentistry)**
Independent Nutritional Consultant, Lafayette, Indiana, USA

NICHOLE F. HUNTLEY, MS, PhD
Mazuri Exotic Animal Nutrition, PMI Nutrition International, Arden Hills, Minnesota, USA

CAYLA ISKE, PhD
Omaha's Henry Doorly Zoo & Aquarium, Omaha, Nebraska, USA

ELIZABETH A. KOUTSOS, PhD
EnviroFlight, LLC, Apex, North Carolina, USA

Y. BECCA LEUNG, BSc, BVSc, PhD
Diplomate, American College of Veterinary Internal Medicine; Veterinary Nutrition Group,
Sydney, Australia

SHANNON LIVINGSTON, MSc
Disney's Animals, Science and Environment, Lake Buena Vista, Florida, USA

BREANNA P. MODICA, MS, MPhil
EnviroFlight, LLC, Apex, North Carolina, USA

JENNIFER L. PARSONS, MS, PhD
Nutrition Advisor, Association of Zoos and Aquarium's Rodent-Insectivore-Lagomorph Taxon Advisory Group, Senior Nutritionist, Mazuri Exotic Animal Nutrition, PMI Nutrition International, Arden Hills, Minnesota, USA

KATHLEEN E. SULLIVAN, MS, PhD
Disney's Animals, Science and Environment, Lake Buena Vista, Florida, USA

ALYXANDRA SWANHALL, BS
Disney's Animals, Science and Environment, Lake Buena Vista, Florida, USA

Contents

Rodents represent a diverse group that shares commonalities in approaches to dietary management. Nutritional management of companion rodents must diverge from laboratory animal management, and must also consider the importance of a healthy gastrointestinal microbiome. Published requirements must be applied appropriately to species, life stage, and body condition management. Common nutritional health concerns include digestive-tract dysbiosis, gastrointestinal stasis, dental malocclusion, obesity, and hypervitaminosis D. Health issues may be avoided or alleviated through proactive management of appropriate feedstuffs in correct proportion, avoidance of most feeds made specifically for laboratory rodents, and emphasis on promoting healthy activity through environmental enrichment.

Proper nutrition and feeding management are the foundation of good health. Nutrition is one area the veterinary health care team can affect. Optimal feeding practices of companion birds are constantly being evaluated. It is critical that health care team members understand the key nutritional factors in avian nutrition, as this allows for the proper recommendation and education of nutrition to bird owners. Depending on the species, today's pet birds may live decades, so it is imperative that proper nutrition habits be adopted by the owner for their avian pet. Educating the owner on proper nutrition and prevention of obesity is one of the most important roles of the veterinary health care team.

It is understood that ferrets are obligate carnivores. Constraints of manufacturing and cost make it difficult to align a single commercial diet to meet all physiological needs of ferrets. Thus, a combination of dietary formats should be offered. Ferret diets should be high in protein and fat and low in carbohydrates. Emphasis should be placed on fat concentrations and protein-to-fat ratios, which can be targeted at 2:1. Plant-based ingredients do not have a place in ferret diets and could unbalance diets, particularly in amino acids. Items such as fruits, while highly palatable to ferrets, should be avoided.

Insectivores are represented in virtually all taxa, although more is known about mammalian and avian insectivore nutrition than for reptiles, amphibia and fish. Establishing nutrient requirements is challenging but recommendations should be based on data from similar taxa, similar GI tract physiology, and known nutritional concerns. In order to provide an appropriate diet for insectivores, consideration must be given to anatomy and method for procuring insects in free-ranging habitats, availability of feeder insects and the resulting dietary nutrient profiles, and complementing those profiles with appropriate diet items from various other categories including formulated feed, produce, animal matter, seeds or grains etc. Consideration of known nutritional concerns for a given species, and the variation in energy requirements in a captively managed situation are essential.

Evidence-based recommendations for the amount, type, and frequency of food items and supplements are lacking for bearded dragons. General recommendations based on ecological data, a few studies, and experts in the field are to: provide at least 50% high-fiber plant matter dusted in pure calcium and less than 50% adult and lower fat larval insects gut loaded with an 8% calcium diet and dusted with pure calcium, provide ultraviolet B lighting for vitamin D3 synthesis, provide multivitamins on a weekly basis, or monthly at minimum, provide a water dish large enough to soak and drink.

Chelonian nutrition is still a young, but very important field of study. This article provides practical feeding advice for tortoises and freshwater and terrestrial turtles. Areas covered include the different feeding ecology of different types of chelonians, their digestive physiology, growth rate, body condition scoring, an overview of what types of diets items can be used in captive diets, and examples of diets used for various species of chelonians.

Mini pigs are engaging, intelligent animals that require different management than other pet species. Published nutrient requirements for production pigs are a good reference, but they must be critically evaluated in the context of pet mini pigs' needs to prioritize longevity and healthy weight. A balanced diet includes a pelleted feed, vegetables, and roughage, with minimal fruit or other treats. Mini pigs easily gain weight, and a balanced, high-fiber diet helps maintain healthy body condition to reduce the risk of metabolic and joint diseases.

Y. Becca Leung

Malnutrition is a known concern during hospitalization for humans, dogs, and cats. The same nutrition principals to reduce the risk of malnutrition can be applied to exotic companion animal patients. However, it's important to understand that many nutritional requirements are ill defined for specific species and prudent clinical judgment is required.

Kathleen E. Sullivan, Alyxandra Swanhall, and Shannon Livingston

Serum micronutrient analysis can provide insight into diet and clinical assessment, despite the complicated interplay between micronutrients and species idiosyncrasies. Approach serum nutrient analytes with skepticism, before jumping to alter diets or offering supplementation. Utilize across species but know that some exotics have exceptions to typical ranges, such as calcium in rabbits or iron in reptiles. Make sure you trust that referenced ranges reflect normal and healthy for that species. Micronutrients are integral to every bodily process, so measurement of serum analytes can tell a story that aids in the clinical picture, when one can recognize what stands out.

VETERINARY CLINICS OF NORTH AMERICA: EXOTIC ANIMAL PRACTICE

SERIES OF RELATED INTEREST

Veterinary Clinics: Small Animal Practice
https://www.vetsmall.theclinics.com/
Advances in Small Animal Care
https://www.advancesinsmallanimalcare.com

THE CLINICS ARE NOW AVAILABLE ONLINE!
Access your subscription at:
www.theclinics.com

Preface

Staying Current—It Takes a Village

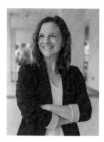

Amanda J. Ardente, DVM, PhD
Editor

Nutrition and husbandry have always been essential considerations for veterinarians and the health care teams seeing exotic companion animals in clinical practice. The field of comparative animal nutrition, specifically for exotic species, continues to evolve as we improve our understanding of species' natural history, unique physiology, energy, and nutrient needs. We are also obtaining more complete nutrient information on food items fed, learning how various nutrients interact, and better understanding how laboratory analyses impact our decision-making process. All this active research means that we need to keep current with the literature to help us optimize the nutritional health of the animals under our care.

So, when the opportunity presented itself to act as managing editor for this Nutrition issue, I could not pass it up. As a veterinarian and nutritionist that specializes in exotic species, this assignment was right up my alley. Our colleagues, who graciously contributed to this work, include boarded specialists in zoologic medicine and in veterinary nutrition, credentialed veterinary technician specialists in nutrition, and doctorate-level comparative nutritionists, working in academia, zoos, and the feed industry. I felt it essential to include these varied, impressive educational and experiential backgrounds because as scientific professionals, we are all committed to a lifetime of learning and can learn so much from each other; I certainly did as I read through these articles prior to their publication.

With back-to-back appointments, full exam rooms, and clients waiting in the lobby, obtaining thorough diet histories may not be prioritized. If you are fortunate enough to gather the information, you still must know or be able to find—quickly—the most important nutrient-related considerations for that species and assess if the diet fed is appropriate. Having textbooks within reach, like these nutrition issues of the *Veterinary Clinics of North America: Exotic Animal Practice* series, makes that job easier. In this text, articles, such as "Insectivore Nutrition - A Review of Current Knowledge" and "Key Nutritional Factors and Obesity Prevention in Companion Psittacine Birds," are

Vet Clin Exot Anim 27 (2024) ix–x
https://doi.org/10.1016/j.cvex.2023.09.001
1094-9194/24/© 2023 Published by Elsevier Inc.

particularly useful for ensuring that your diet recommendations are current and practical as a part of your preventative health plan. On the other hand, if during your patient examination, you find the animal to be in poor body condition, lethargic, or described with inappetence, articles like "Interpretation of Serum Analytes for Nutritional Evaluation" and "Assisted Enteral Feeding of Exotic Companion Animals" will help you devise a diagnostic plan to determine whether poor nutrition led to clinical or subclinical disease and develop an appropriate treatment plan.

I certainly hope that you enjoy this issue, covering a wide range of topics from rodents, to bearded dragons, to miniature pigs, and find it useful in your practice. To all the authors who took time out of their busy schedules, we appreciate your commitment to bettering our patient care for these exotic companion animals and sincerely thank you for your contribution! It certainly takes a village to ensure that we continue improving upon the incorporation of nutrition into our veterinary practice.

Amanda J. Ardente, DVM, PhD
Ardente Veterinary Nutrition LLC
Ocala, FL, USA

E-mail address:
amanda@ardentevetnutrition.com

Nutritional Physiology and Feeding of Companion Rodents

Jennifer L. Parsons, MS, PhD[a,b,*]

KEYWORDS

- Rodent • Rat • Mouse • Hamster • Guinea pig • Chinchilla • Nutrition • Microbiome
- Digestive tract

KEY POINTS

- Feeding to each species' dietary niche is paramount, because not all rodents share the same evolutionary history; diets should be adjusted to species accordingly.
- Dietary health issues for many rodents stem from the historic tendency to model all rodent diets after those suited for domestic rats and mice, whose physiology and nutritional ecology differ significantly from most other rodent species.
- Historic rodent diets were also modeled for the needs of laboratory animal applications, which similarly differ significantly from the needs of companion animals.
- A focus on the health of the digestive tract microbiome is extremely important, including provision of proper substrates (foodstuffs as well as water), and support for species-appropriate cecotrophy.
- Unique nutritional health needs of rodents include management for near-continual foraging, constant incisor growth, and unique vitamin requirements for some species.

BACKGROUND

Nutritional Ecology

Members of order Rodentia share many similarities in appearance as well as feeding habits. To effectively manage their dietary husbandry, an understanding of the role of diet niche, evolutionary history, and free-ranging ecology is important. Almost all rodents worldwide are foragers on primarily plant matter, within a range of categories: specialist herbivores, generalist herbivores, granivores, omnivores, frugivores, and (represented by a small handful of species) insectivores. Companion rodents fall almost entirely into the first 4 of these categories. Specialist herbivores consume

[a] Association of Zoos and Aquarium's Rodent-Insectivore-Lagomorph Taxon Advisory Group;
[b] Mazuri Exotic Animal Nutrition, PMI Nutrition International, 4001 Lexington Avenue North, Arden Hills, MN 55126, USA
* Corresponding author.
E-mail address: jparsons@mazuri.com

Vet Clin Exot Anim 27 (2024) 1–12
https://doi.org/10.1016/j.cvex.2023.08.001
1094-9194/24/© 2023 Elsevier Inc. All rights reserved.

vetexotic.theclinics.com

mainly monocots (grasses), forbs, and shrubs; generalist herbivores consume similar items to specialist herbivores, with partial or seasonal reliance on additional feeds such as seeds, nuts, or fruiting bodies.[1] Omnivores expand the diet of a generalist herbivore to include animal matter such as insects, and granivores subsist on a majority seed diet.[1] It is important to note here that, with very few exceptions, wild-type fruits, seeds/nuts, and other categories of foodstuffs differ significantly in nutritional composition from analogs cultivated by humans (**Tables 1** and **2**).

Most rodents consume extremely high-fiber diets and derive a large amount of dietary energy from the digestion of either plant fiber (plant cell wall components), or cell solubles (enzymes and other molecules located inside the plant cell).[2] Plant fiber is made up of 3 types of molecules, which differ in proportion with plant type and part: (1) hemicellulose, which is partially digestible by mammalian enzymes, (2) cellulose, which no vertebrate enzymes can break down but which can be digested by microbial enzymes, and (3) lignin, which is completely indigestible.[2,3] Herbivores that consume high-cellulose diets usually develop extensive anatomic and metabolic adaptations to host large populations of symbiotic microbes within their gastrointestinal tract and to utilize the metabolites synthesized by these microbes during cellulose digestion.[2,3]

Digestive Anatomy and Physiology

Vertebrates adapted to utilize dietary cellulose diverge into 2 main groups: foregut fermenters and hindgut fermenters. Foregut or pregastric fermenters have developed specialized outpouchings of the esophagus, and ingested feed passes through sometimes extensive compartments before the true (glandular) stomach.[2,4] These compartments host a diverse and complex ecosystem of cellulolytic protozoa, bacteria, fungi, and yeast.[2,4] Hindgut fermenters host a similar microcosm within the intestinal tract instead, with extensive development and specialization of structures distal to the small intestine.[2,4] Virtually all rodents are hindgut fermenters to some degree (**Fig. 1**).[4] Although the colon is the primary site for cellulose digestion in many large-bodied

Table 1
Nutrient composition comparison among major categories of produce and forage, along with wild-type fruits

| Nutrient, % of Dry Matter | Wild Fruits | Commercial Produce | | | | Grasses (Hay) | Alfalfa Hay |
		Fruits	Starchy Vegetables[a]	Other Vegetables	Greens		
Protein	12.1	3.7	5.8	17.1	22.9	11.1	18.0
Acid-detergent fiber	37.2	6.6	6.9	12.1	12.4	33.4	29.6
Neutral-detergent fiber	48.2	12.1	14.9	28.6	17.3	65.4	
Sugars	7.6	17.1	12.4	30.5	10.2	9.3	
Starches	1.7	64.5	40.6	19.6	14.3	4.3	
Calcium	0.88	0.04	0.20	0.26	1.02	0.54	1.3
Phosphorus	0.23	0.08	0.21	0.45	0.40	0.20	0.23

[a] Includes root vegetables, corn, winter squashes, and peas.
Mean data from Kendrick EL, Shipley LA, Hagerman AE, Kelley LM. Fruit and fiber: The nutritional value of figs for a small tropical ruminant, the blue duiker (*Cephalophus monticola*). Afr. J. Ecol. 2009; 47:556 to 566; U.S. Department of Agriculture, Agricultural Research Service. National Nutrient Database for Standard Reference. 2016; National Research Council. Nutrient Requirements of Horses. 6th rev ed. The National Academies Press; 2007.

Table 2
Nutrient composition comparison among wild-type and cultivated nuts and seeds

Nutrient, %	Baobab Seed	Wild-type Nuts	Peanuts	Sunflower Seeds	Almonds	Walnuts	Macadamia	Millet
Protein	36.3	8.0	25.7	22.8	20.0	24.4	8.3	11.0
Crude fiber	14.1		8.5	8.6	12.5	6.8	8.6	8.5
Fat	29.3	5.3	49.2	49.6	52.2	56.6	73.7	4.2
Calcium		1.0	0.06	0.12	0.27	0.06	0.07	0.01
Phosphorus		0.9	0.38	0.70	0.52	0.46	0.14	0.29

Mean data from Murray SS, Schoeninger MJ, Bunn HT, Pickering TR, Marlett JA. Nutritional composition of some wild plant foods and honey used by Hadza foragers of Tanzania. J Food Compost Anal 2001; 14(1):3 to 13; Agrahar-Murugkar D, Subbulakshmi G. Nutritive values of wild edible fruits, berries, nuts, roots and spices consumed by the Khasi tribes of India. Ecol Food Nutr 2005; 44:207 to 223; U.S. Department of Agriculture, Agricultural Research Service. National Nutrient Database for Standard Reference. 2016

hindgut fermenters (eg, equids), rodents in particular show significant specialization of the cecum, where the majority of microbial activity occurs in these species.[4] A handful of exceptions exist, because some rodents (eg, hamsters) have developed a combination of foregut and hindgut fermentation, with a pregastric region in the stomach, which houses a microbial population, lower pH than the glandular portion of the

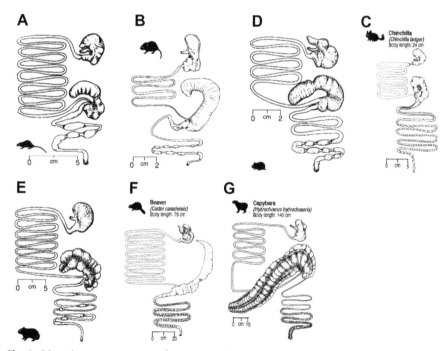

Fig. 1. Digestive tract anatomy of representative companion and wild rodent species, in order of increasing anatomical and physiological complexity from left to right and top to bottom. (A) Domestic rat, (B) hamster, (C) vole, (D) chinchilla, (E) guinea pig, (F) beaver, and (G) capybara. *Adapted from* Stevens CE, Hume ID. Comparative Physiology of the Vertebrate Digestive System. 2nd ed. Cambridge University Press; 1995, with permission.

stomach, and similar function to the rumen in both fermentation and dietary urea utilization (**Fig. 2**).[2,4,5]

Due to the ability of gut microbes to convert cellulose into useful metabolites, microbial cells themselves represent an important source of nutrition. As microbes live out their normal life cycle and die, they pass out of the principal fermentation chamber to mingle with ingesta. Foregut fermenters digest these cells in the glandular stomach, whereas cecal fermenters can form discrete masses of microbial cells within the cecum, packaged within a layer of mucus to avoid comingling with colon contents as they travel distally: these "packets" are called cecotropes.[6] Through neural signaling from the hind end, cecal fermenters are alerted to cecotropes about to pass, and will consume them directly from the anus, thus recovering a significant amount of nutrients that would otherwise be lost in feces.[6] This process is called cecotrophy (differentiated from coprophagy, which describes consumption of feces or undigested feed, rather than cecotropes[6]), and is quite well documented in rabbits as well; lagomorphs and many rodents that are prevented from practicing cecotrophy will develop nutritional deficiencies.[7]

Proper maintenance of the microbial environment is crucial to any animal that depends on energy from cellulolysis. Microbes require a consistent source of fuel (in this case, cellulose), consistency regarding pH, temperature, and fluid volume, and time for gradual adaptation to any change in environment.[2] Microbial communities respond to change through microevolution: altering proportions of microbe species during the course of several generations. Thus, a sudden change in dietary substrates will lead to either inefficient feed breakdown or a suboptimal environment for the microbial species present at that moment.[2]

Microbial fermentation produces 3 main byproducts: volatile fatty acids (VFAs), acidic compounds (eg, lactic acid), and gas (CO_2 and CH_4).[2] Foregut and hindgut fermenters use VFAs as an energy source, and the structural properties of their digestive tract allow passage of these short-chain molecules into the bloodstream and on to the liver for further metabolism.[2,3] Under ideal conditions, production of gas and

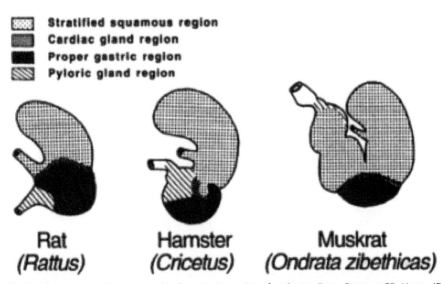

Fig. 2. Distribution of gastric epithelium in 3 species of rodents. *From* Stevens CE, Hume ID Comparative Physiology of the Vertebrate Digestive System. 2nd ed. Cambridge University Press; 1995.,with permission.

acids is minimal; however, when overexposed to easily-digested and rapidly-fermented substrates, runaway fermentation can occur, causing digestive-tract acidosis and gas build-up. This condition is described as rumenoacidosis or bloat in foregut fermenters, and colitis or colic in hindgut fermenters.[2] Colic poses structural hazards (distention and intestinal perforation), as well as the risk of acidosis extending to the bloodstream and setting off further metabolic derangements.[2] Low hindgut pH begins to kill resident microbes, which can release toxins as they die off. These toxins can also enter the bloodstream, where they often lodge in regions of poor vascularization and cause tissue necrosis, a condition called laminitis in equids and similar species.[2] Hindgut fermenters are somewhat shielded from the effects of rapidly-fermentable dietary substrates, compared with foregut fermenters, by the placement of their microbial community at the end of the tract, after much has been digested and absorbed in the glandular stomach and small intestine. However, heavy loads of easily-fermentable compounds, especially those to which the animal is not accustomed, can still reach the hindgut.

Rodents and lagomorphs are known for their continuously-growing incisors, ostensibly an adaptation to constantly chewing on tough plant material, or forages with a high-silica content.[8] Under human care, animals without hard materials to chew on can quickly develop dental overgrowth and malocclusions, which impair normal dietary intake. Hard substrates can be provided, either in the diet or in the form of non-toxic wood blocks or similar commercially-sold products, with a preference toward the latter, because most hard pellets are rarely formulated for the species under discussion (as will be expained in depthlater in this article).

Rodents have several unique needs related to their typically diminutive nature as well, especially when coupled with their aforementioned gastrointestinal anatomy and nutritional ecology. Small body size results in a large surface area to volume ratio, creating substantial mass-specific energetic demands.[9] Free-ranging rodents therefore evolved high metabolic rates, and spend the majority of their waking hours foraging, with near-constant ingestion of often fibrous plant matter. Thus, much of their nutritional physiology is adapted to continual throughput of ingesta, and even in domesticity, these taxa require frequent feed intake for proper digestive function and metabolism, as well as to maintain the gut microbial community.[7]

Key Nutritional Factors

Energy

Energy requirements have not been quantified for most rodent species. For the laboratory rat, maintenance energy intake of 112 $kcal/BW_{kg}^{0.75}$ seems sufficient, with the gestation requirement between 10% and 30% greater than those for maintenance (depending on litter size and phase of gestation), and the lactation requirement at least 311 $kcal/BW_{kg}^{0.75}$, again depending on litter size.[7] For the laboratory mouse, sufficient energy intake for maintenance was estimated at 161 $kcal ME/BW_{kg}^{0.75}$, for gestation at up to 360 $kcal ME/BW_{kg}^{0.75}$, and for peak lactation at 310 to 430 $kcal ME/BW_{kg}^{0.75}$ for large litters.[7] For both species, energy needs for growth were not possible to estimate completely without sufficient information about the animal, its activity level, and environment.[7] However, one could expect that energy needs would lie between those for maintenance and reproduction.

For other rodent species, energy needs of rats and mice could be used as a starting place to estimate total feed intake; however, for all rodents (including rats and mice), it is essential to adjust feed intake based on body condition, especially considering differences in efficiency of feed digestion among species, life stages, and individual animals.

Water

Appropriate water intake is not only essential to an animal's basic physiologic and cellular functions but in the presence of significant gut microbial communities, the maintenance of proper fluid volume in the gastrointestinal lumen also ensures a healthy microbiome.[2] Therefore, ensuring free access to clean, fresh water that is ideally near room temperature is paramount. Many rodents may be acclimated to use an inverted drinkers fitted with ball valves, diaphragm-style valves, or similar attachments, and this provides the most effective way to ensure continual access to clean water—provided the reservoir is cleaned and refilled ideally daily.

Protein

For species that rely on microbial fermentation for adequate digestion, microbial cells represent an important pool of high-quality protein, with optimal amino-acid balance. For rodent species that routinely practice cecotrophy, ensuring a balanced diet requires free access to this important nutrient source. Once species-appropriate access to microbial protein is ensured, dietary protein needs fall along diet niche lines (**Tables 3** and **4**). Excess protein can represent a significant substrate for excessively-rapid microbial fermentation, leading to the suite of gut health issues mentioned above and below. Therefore, for best digestive tract health, it is generally recommended to feed toward the lower end of recommended protein ranges (see **Table 4**) for animals at maintenance, and toward the higher end of these ranges for animals undergoing reproduction or juvenile growth.

Fat

Few studies exist to quantify total lipid requirements for rodents, apart from quantities that ensure rapid growth and/or reproduction in high-producing laboratory colonies. Given the need to manage body condition to ensure long-term health, more moderate dietary fat levels are recommended, again varying slightly by diet niche (see **Table 4**).

Carbohydrates

Plant cellulose in the form of dietary fiber is an essential substrate for gastrointestinal microbiota, and an important source of energy in the form of VFAs; proper provision of dietary fiber (see **Table 4**) is extremely important to rodent health. Equally as important is the control of sugars and starches, which represent extremely readily-fermentable substrates and can lead to significant dysbiosis. Sugar intake must be minimized as much as possible, and an appropriate balance must be struck between

Table 3
Published nutrient requirements for laboratory rodents

Nutrient, % of As-fed Diet	Granivores: Domestic Rat/Mouse		Specialist Herbivore: Guinea Pig (Growth)	Specialist Herbivore: Vole (Growth)	Omnivore: Hamster (Growth and Reproduction)
	Growth	Maintenance			
Protein	15–18	5	18	11–13	16–18
Fat	5	5			3–5
Fiber		<7	13–15	25	
Calcium	0.5		0.8		0.6–1.0
Phosphorus	0.3		0.4		0.4–0.7
Vit C (mg/kg)	N/A	N/A	200	N/A	N/A

Data from National Research Council. Nutrient Requirements of Laboratory Animals. 4th rev ed. The National Academies Press; 1995

Table 4
Appropriate total-diet nutrient concentrations for representative rodents, by diet niche

	Domestic Mice/Rats	Generalist/Omnivorous Rodents (Chinchilla, Hamster, Gerbil)	Herbivorous Rodents (Guinea Pig, Vole)
Protein (%)	15–20	14–20	10–18
Crude fiber (%)	<7	10–15	>20
Lipid (%)	5–7	3–5	2–3
Starch (%)	10–20	< 10	<10
Calcium (%)	0.5–1.0	0.5–1.0	0.5–1.0
Phosphorus (%)	0.3–0.5	0.3–0.5	0.3–0.5
Vit D (IU/kg)	1000–1500	1000–1500	1000–1500
Vit C (mg/kg)	N/A	N/A	200–300[a]

[a] For cavies (growth requirement).

dietary starch and fiber, based on the evolutionary history of the species in question (see **Table 4**). For strictly herbivorous rodents in particular (such as guinea pigs), dietary starches should be minimized and dietary fiber emphasized as much as possible.

Vitamins
Yet another benefit of microbial fermentation is the production of all known B vitamins as well as vitamin K in the regions of the digestive tract where it occurs.[2] However, the hindgut does not absorb vitamins well, thereby making cecotrophy especially important to the satisfaction of micronutrient requirements.

Fat-soluble vitamins A and E are dietary essentials for all rodents. For vitamin A, most species seem to have similar requirements at 2400 IU/kg diet.[7] Vitamin E requirements depend on the form of tocopherol used: Research with rats and mice has found that RRR-α-tocopherol works best with these species, with a similar requirement for both species of 18 to 22 mg/kg diet, or 27 to 32 IU/kg diet.[7] Other forms of tocopherol may be used but dose must be scaled to biological activity. Of note is the possibility for selenium status to influence dietary vitamin E needs because these 2 nutrients may interact with each other. Thus, a selenium-deficient animal may need higher amounts of vitamin E; conversely, an excess of either nutrient may reduce needs for the other or could even induce toxicity.

Vitamin D_3 requirements also seem similar across rodent species and are currently estimated at 1000 IU/kg of diet.[7] It is particularly important to note here that most free-ranging rodents are crepuscular or spend a significant amount of time in burrows or under heavy forest canopy. These species have naturally low requirements for vitamin D and can develop hypervitaminosis quite quickly when exposed to large amounts of exogenous synthetic vitamin D_3. High-quality rodent feeds are formulated with this lower requirement in mind, and generalized herbivore feeds typically contain reasonably moderate amounts of D_3. However, care must be taken to avoid inadvertent consumption of feeds made for other species—especially those intended for primates, whose vitamin D_3 requirements are considerably higher. Similar to the other fat-soluble vitamins mentioned above, vitamin D_3 in excess can become toxic quite quickly, and historically (and at times still today), hypervitaminosis D in rodents was and is common and often dramatic[10] and can result in metastatic calcification of soft tissues across a range of presentations, with the location and severity of lesions depending on both species and dose.

Unlike most mammals, members of the family Caviidae (cavies and maras) cannot synthesize ascorbic acid (vitamin C) quickly enough to meet nutritional requirements,[7] a trait shared by a sporadic group including primates, dolphins, vampire bats, and some fish. Domestic guinea pigs must therefore be provided with a source of vitamin C, either via fortified feeds or via a variety of water-soluble products in their drinking water.

Finally, it should be noted that vitamins, particularly those in the fat-soluble category, may interact with each other. Oftentimes, an excess of one vitamin may express as a deficiency in another—for example, hypervitaminosis E can present as hypovitaminosis K, or hypervitaminosis A may express as hypovitaminosis D or E. In cases where an excess or deficiency of a given vitamin is suspected, analysis of other vitamins that may potentially interact is highly recommended.

Another important note with vitamins regards the choice of analytical method, and practitioners should never be afraid to discuss laboratory methods and sensitivities with contract laboratories. In general, chromatographic techniques (gas chromatography or liquid chromatography) work best for vitamins, and radioimmunoassay or enzyme-linked immunosorbent assay-based methods tend to lack accuracy and/or repeatability.

Minerals

Rodents also seem to share similar mineral requirements across taxa, and those published for the laboratory rat and mouse may suffice for other species. Calcium and phosphorus are of particular interest, with animals at maintenance requiring lower dietary concentrations than those undergoing growth or reproduction (see **Tables 3** and **4**). Because these nutrients interact with each other, total-diet calcium intake must be greater than that for phosphorus, in a generally-recommended ratio of 1.5 to 2:1 Ca:P.[7] Calcium and phosphorus also depend on vitamin D_3 for regulation of absorption and metabolism, and deficiency or toxicity signs can be very similar; therefore, analysis of all 3 nutrients is highly recommended when investigating a suspected deficiency or excess in 1 of the 3.

Less is known about other mineral requirements in rodent species, but again domestic rat and mouse literature may be consulted as a starting point.[7] As in all mammals, magnesium and potassium may interact with each other and also with calcium and/or phosphorus; therefore, care must be taken to choose well-balanced feeds, and again a full mineral panel may be useful when diagnosing suspected mineral issues. Similarly, copper, iron, and zinc may inhibit each other, and as mentioned previously, selenium and vitamin E may interact. Fortunately, laboratory methodology is much more standardized with regard to minerals than for vitamins, and most reputable contract laboratories return reliable, affordable results.

Other Nutritional Health Concerns

Great care should be taken regarding management and maintenance of a healthy digestive tract, especially given the complex interactions among the gut microbial community and the host animal's own digestive anatomy and physiology. As mentioned previously, improper proportions of dietary fiber and easily-fermentable carbohydrates can lead to chronic colitis (and associated follow-on pathology) or acute colic. Interruptions in feed intake can cause a simple energy deficiency or, when combined with insufficient hydration, can cause gastrointestinal stasis, a dysfunction in the normal mechanisms for peristalsis, and a slow-down in passage rate.[11] Animals that either are fasted too long or undergo voluntary hyporexia or anorexia could experience a shutdown of cecal function as microbes are depleted of fuel and die off en masse.[11] In clinical cases where gastrointestinal microbiome has been severely disrupted, normal function may in some cases be restored through fecal microbial transplantation from a healthy conspecific that has been screened for internal parasites and other infectious disease.

Because rodents are very efficient with digestion and nutrient assimilation, obesity is a problem in individuals under human care that do not experience the temperature demands and activity levels of wild counterparts. Obesity poses the same health risks as with all mammalian species but additionally restricts animals from effectively practicing cecotrophy. Until the obesity is resolved, it is important to ensure that the base of the animal's enclosure is solid (not wire mesh), to allow it to find and consume cecotropes. Obesity is challenging to manage in these species because the solutions common to other animals (limit-feeding or meal-feeding) risk complications from inconsistent passage of ingesta.

RECOMMENDATIONS

To prevent nutritional issues, consideration of each species' dietary niche and the needs of their microbial population is important. Diet item choices must be tailored accordingly: high-fiber, low-sugar, low-starch diets for specialist herbivores, with somewhat higher starches and lower fiber permissible for granivores and omnivores. **Table 4** summarizes total-diet nutrient recommendations for representative species by diet niche.

For virtually all species, produce is not an ideal diet foundation: on a dry-matter basis, commercial produce is low in fiber, high in protein, and in the case of fruit, extremely high in sugars (see **Table 1**). Fruit is almost never an appropriate diet item for rodent species, and for the most specialized herbivores such as guinea pigs, it is recommended to avoid fruit completely. Small amounts of low-starch produce such as dark greens or nonstarchy vegetables may be allowed in rodent diets for husbandry reasons (eg, training, medication vehicles), but for all rodent species it is recommended to feed produce in controlled, measured quantities, in smaller proportions relative to forages and/or fortified feeds that provide fiber.

For specialist and generalist herbivores (eg, guinea pig and chinchilla), consistent intake of forage (grasses) is important. These species do best when fed a diet similar to large-bodied grazing herbivores: freely available grass hay and a quality high-fiber pellet—although generalist herbivores also may do well on reduced quantities of hay if provided with sufficient fiber in the fortified portion of the diet. Alfalfa hay is not appropriate for animals at maintenance, and although it may be used with breeding, growing, or senior animals, it should be given only in very limited and measured quantities, because it is generally too high in protein, calcium, and easily-fermented nutrients (see **Table 1**). Pellets should ideally contain more than 20% crude fiber and less than 10% starch; this was once difficult to find in commercial feeds but with recent advances in manufacturing technology, low-starch commercial pellets are now available.

The temptation often arises with many companion rodent owners to feed a seed-based or nut-based diet; however, for reasons similar to the previous discussion of commercial produce, providing significant quantities of seeds or nuts should be avoided. As with human-cultivated produce, commercially-available seeds and nuts share little resemblance to wild-type seeds, and are much lower in fiber, higher in fat, and depleted of essential nutrients (see **Table 2**). Such products contribute to obesity and can cause nutritional deficiencies, especially in calcium: they naturally lack calcium, and excessive fats may bind calcium in the gastrointestinal tract, creating calcium soaps that evade digestion and absorption.[12] Seeds or nuts may again be offered as occasional tools to encourage foraging behavior or for other husbandry needs but should be restricted to lower-fat options and fed in very limited quantities.

Because the field of rodent nutrition was initially orientated heavily toward laboratory animal care, caution should be exercised when selecting feeds for rodents in particular. The first (and still many) commercial feed labeled for rodents was developed to meet nutritional profiles suited for laboratory mice and rats, 2 extreme granivores bred from wild counterparts that evolved in close association with human habitation and human granaries. Domestic rats and mice are therefore adapted to higher-starch, higher-protein, and lower-fiber diets than the majority of rodent species. Laboratory rodent feeds can also be heavily fortified with vitamin D_3 to meet the needs of indoor colonies intended for reproduction. Therefore, "rodent pellets" are not recommended for specialist or generalist herbivores, and one should instead search for species-appropriate options—especially in the case of guinea pigs, which not only require a very high-fiber and low-starch diet but also require feeds fortified with vitamin C. However, when feeding truly granivorous species under indoor conditions, quality fortified feed intended for domestic rats and mice may form the basis of a healthy diet.

Management of obesity while ensuring consistent feed intake requires a number of approaches. Rodents can efficiently utilize poor-quality feed sources, so simply switching an animal to a "low-calorie" (high-fiber) diet as one would with a dog or human will not suffice. Slow feeders or puzzle feeders may be used to slow intake and draw out the time it takes to consume a given amount of calories; they may also provide mental stimulation, which is important for any animal under human care. When further limitation of dietary calories becomes difficult, energy expenditure can be increased by providing ample opportunity for physical activity. Some animals may be trained to walk in a harness, and several products exist that encourage rodents to move and explore. However, when selecting a form of exercise such as a wheel or ball, great care should be taken to ensure that animal welfare best practices are met, with regard to the size and shape of the device relative to the animal's form, the safe functioning of the device, and avoidance of mental stress—for example, by exposing an unacclimated prey species to situations that simulate predation.

SUMMARY

Rodents represent a diverse group of species across a range of evolutionary backgrounds, which nonetheless share commonalities in approaches to dietary management. Nutritional management of companion rodents must diverge from laboratory animal management and must consider the importance of a healthy gastrointestinal microbiome to successful animal health outcomes. Where published nutrient requirements exist, they must be applied appropriately to species, life stage, and body-condition management, and extrapolation of requirements from similar species should be done with care. Common nutritional health concerns include digestive tract dysbiosis, gastrointestinal stasis, dental malocclusion, obesity, and hypervitaminosis D. These and other concerns may be avoided or alleviated through proactive management of appropriate feedstuffs in correct proportion, avoidance of most feeds made specifically for laboratory rodents, and emphasis on promoting healthy physical activity levels and mental stimulation through environmental enrichment.

CLINICS CARE POINTS

- Proper diet management consists of diet-niche-appropriate balance of macronutrients, provision of vitamin-fortified and mineral-fortified feeds, species-appropriate freedom to exercise cecotrophy, and free access to clean water.
- Digestive-tract dysbiosis may be avoided and/or potentially corrected by establishing the right dietary balance of fiber, sugars/starches, and protein. Fecal microbial transplant may be a powerful tool to recover significantly disturbed microbiome.
- Unique considerations for the management of rodent nutritional health include their small body size (and therefore high metabolic rate and need to eat continuously), ever-growing incisors, and specific nutrient needs such as vitamin C for cavies.
- Obesity can be challenging to manage and can present add-on health issues; body condition is more easily managed proactively, through careful selection of diet items and encouragement of activity via environmental enrichment.
- In cases of suspected micronutrient excess or deficiency, multinutrient analyses are highly recommended. In the case of vitamins, choice of laboratory and analytical method are extremely important.

DISCLOSURE

Dr J.L. Parsons is a nutritionist with Mazuri Exotic Animal Nutrition, which markets rodent products.

REFERENCES

1. Parsons JL. Nitrogen requirements of Southern Plains small mammals: dietary niche, life history, and environmental implications, . Thesis. Stillwater, OK: Oklahoma State University; 2001.
2. Pond WG, Church DC, Pond KR, et al. Basic animal nutrition and feeding. 5th edition. Hoboken, NJ: Wiley; 2005.
3. Robbins CT. Wildlife feeding and nutrition. 2nd edition. San Diego, CA: Academic Press; 2001.
4. Stevens CE, Hume ID. Comparative physiology of the vertebrate digestive system. 2nd edition. New York, NY: Cambridge University Press; 1995.
5. Reznik G, Reznik-Schuller H, Mohr U. Clinical anatomy of the European hamster *Cricetus cricetus* L. U.S. Government Printing Office; 1978. Available at: https://digital. library.unt.edu/ark:/67531/metadc28308/m1/163/?q=proventriculus. Accessed March 10, 2023.
6. Guerra Aldrigui L, Gama Nogueira-Filho SL, Mendes A, et al. Effect of different feeding regimes on cecotrophy behavior and retention of solute and particle markers in the digestive tract of paca (*Cunniculus paca*). Comp Biochem Physiol A 2018;226:57–65.
7. National Research Council. Nutrient requirements of laboratory animals. 4th rev edition. Washington, DC: The National Academies Press; 1995.
8. Martin LF, Ackermans NL, Tollefson TN, et al. Tooth wear, growth and height in rabbits (Oryctolagus cuniculus) fed pelleted or extruded diets with or without added abrasives. J Anim Physiol Anim Nutr (Berl) 2022;106(3):630–41.
9. McNab BK. The physiological ecology of vertebrates: a view from energetics. Ithaca, NY: Comstock Publishing Associates; 2002.

10. Kenny D, Cambre RC, Lewandowski A, et al. Suspected vitamin D3 toxicity in pacas (*Cuniculus paca*) and agoutis (*Dasyprocta aguti*). J Zoo Wildl Med 1993;24(2):129–39.
11. Harkness JE, Wagner JE. Biology and medicine of rabbits and rodents. 4th edition. York, PA: Williams & Wilkins; 1995.
12. Frommelt L, Bielohuby M, Stoehr BJM, et al. Effects of low-carbohydrate, high-fat diets on apparent digestibility of minerals and trace elements in rats. Nutrition 2014;30(7–8):869–75.

Key Nutritional Factors and Obesity Prevention in Companion Psittacine Birds

Kara M. Burns, MS, MEd, LVT, VTS (Nutrition)

KEYWORDS

• Avian • Psittacine • Nutrition • Obesity • Weight management • Key nutrients

INTRODUCTION

One area of veterinary medicine that affects every pet that comes into the hospital, including companion birds, is nutrition. There are 3 components that affect the life of an animal—genetics, environment, and nutrition. Health is directly correlated to quality of life and life span of the avian species. Nutrition is the one factor that the veterinary health care team can easily affect. Proper nutrition and feeding management are the foundation on which healing and the maintenance of health rests.

Across the globe there are 9000+ avian species.[1] With this wide variety of species, it comes as no surprise that birds have diverse nutritional requirements. Each species of bird has specific nutritional requirements, and this is determined by individual physiology.[2,3] Psittaciformes are frequently referred to as "psittacine birds" and are popular as companion caged pet birds or aviary birds.

Birds within the order Psittaciformes are considered to consume plant-based foodstuffs and are classified as florivores. Within this category, further subclassifications can be made, including granivory (eg, budgies and cockatiels), frugivory (many of the macaws), and nectarivory (eg, lorikeets and lories). In addition to the basic classification based on general foods eaten, ingredients consumed vary over time depending on nutrient availability, gender of the bird, and age.[4]

The veterinary health care team should recognize that nutritional deficiencies or imbalances resulting from primary or secondary disease are common. When evaluating and managing birds, the veterinary team must consider the requirements of the individual species, as well as individual variation due to life stage, lifestyle, and disease conditions. Certain nutritional imbalances lead to specific clinical abnormalities; however, it is imperative for veterinary teams to remember they are only one aspect of a multifactorial quandary.[1] Improper nutrition in a bird may:

- Conceal the true nature of a disease,
- Suppress ability to resist disease,
- Prolong recovery from illness, and
- Decrease reproductive performance.

632 Wexford Drive, Lafayette, IN 47905, USA
E-mail address: karamburns@gmail.com

Vet Clin Exot Anim 27 (2024) 13–29
https://doi.org/10.1016/j.cvex.2023.07.001
1094-9194/24/© 2023 Elsevier Inc. All rights reserved.

Nutritional History

Every bird that presents to the hospital, every time they present, should be assessed to establish nutritional needs and feeding goals, depending on the bird's physiology and health. The veterinary team must perform a patient history and nutritional history, score the patient's body condition, and work together to determine the proper nutritional recommendation for the patient, and communicate this information to the owner.

The first step in evaluating an avian patient and determining its nutritional status is to take a thorough history, including signalment (ie, breed, age, gender, reproductive status). An in-depth nutritional history should be taken every time the avian patient presents to the hospital to determine the quality and adequacy of the food being fed, the feeding protocol (eg, the amount of food given, the family member responsible for feeding, and so forth), the type or types of food given, the bird's activity level, its environment and housing, what is offered at each meal, how often the bird is fed in a day, is it in a cage with another bird, and so on.[5–8]

Veterinary technicians should ask questions to the owner in an open-ended questioning style, thus allowing for the owner to provide reliable and accurate information without suspecting they are being judged by the veterinary team. It also allows owners the opportunity to talk and explain the "what and why" of their actions. A nutritional assessment aids in determining if specific adjustments might be of benefit for the individual patient. The nutritional assessment should also include the bird's body weight in grams and body condition score (BCS). The provision of snacks, treats, and "human" food should be investigated. Similarly, asking owners about how they administer medications can reveal issues not suspected by the owner (eg, vitamin supplements in the patient's drinking water). A nutritional history questionnaire aids the veterinary team in creating a protocol for taking the history of an avian patient (**Fig. 1**).

The information gathered needs to be recorded in the patient's medical record. Every time the patient presents to the hospital, the same questioning process should be repeated. Patients' food habits may change over time alongside what the bird owner provides. In addition, it has been reported that certain species (ie, cockatoos) are able to get owners to feed them only what they want to eat.[6]

It is vital to determine the amount of each food group being consumed by the bird. The food groups used with companion psittacines include fruits, vegetables, protein sources, cereals, and grains including seeds and nuts. In addition, it is important for the veterinary team to ascertain whether and how much balanced nutritional food is consumed. Balanced foods include extruded or pelleted diets or Lafeber's Nutri-Berries and/or Avi-Cakes (Lafeber Company, Cornell, IL, USA). Seed mixes that contain pellets added to balance the formula are not balanced, as birds rarely eat the few added pellets. Thus, nutritional history taking is imperative in determining whether the overall diet is balanced.

Changes in body composition are important concerns in birds and if found, need to be investigated. BCS should be performed, and if possible and without causing undue stress to the avian patient at home, the owner taught to do a BCS. This process allows for the owner to monitor their bird's condition at home and call in to the veterinary team. Ensure the BCS method is consistent to assess changes over time.

BCS is a valuable tool for assessing a patient's general health status and evaluation of a patient's food supply. The BCS system described here is based on scores between 1 and 5, with 1 being emaciated and 5 being obese. As there are numerous avian species, this scoring will be an overarching "broad" system aimed at scoring

Patient information   Date:

Patient name or ID #			
Client name			
Species			
Gender	Determined by DNA__ , Endoscopy__ , Visual__ , Other__		
Hatch Date/Age			
Current BW (g)			
BCS			
Pertinent PE findings			
Medical history			
Current medications:			
Activity level			
	Flighted		Clipped wings

Nutritional History:

Commercial/Formulated Food Fed	Amount fed?	Frequency
Brand		
Form		

Vegetables (be specific)	Amount fed?	Frequency?

Seed Mixtures (be specific)		
Breakfast		
Lunch		
Dinner		
Between meals		
Medications given w/ food or water		
Vitamins or supplements		

Treats - list all types	How much?	How often?

Fig. 1. Avian nutritional assessment form.

companion pet birds. The BCS tool is a subjective assessment of body fat. When scoring, the patient's lifestyle, life stage, and species should be taken into account. An optimal body condition allows for a good overall appearance with a pectoral muscle contour suitable for the species.[9]

To assess body condition, the veterinary team member should (**Fig. 2**) follow the following:

- Palpate the pectoral muscle directly alongside the ventral ridge of the keel bone or carina. Note the convexity or concavity of the pectoral muscle mass contour.

Tell me about your bird's appetite and water intake _____
  Any changes?_____

Where is your bird fed? _____

What time(s) of day is your bird fed?_____

Tell me about medications or supplements given._____
  What is the route of administration? _____

Tell me about any other pets in the home._____

Tell me abut other birds in the home._____

What water supply is provided? __Tap Water ___Bottled Water __ Rain/River Water

Is your bird exposed to sunlight? Y__ N__ Length of time_____ Frequency _____

Does anyone in the home smoke? Y__ N __

Environment:

Housing	Detail	Number
Cage size		
Cage composition		
Bar spacing		
Ventilation space		
Bowl location		
Substrate used to line cage		
Perches		
Toys		
Lighting		
Other		

Fig. 1. (*continued*).

- Note the degree of prominence of the keel.
- Look for subcutaneous fat deposits over the sternum, sides, coelom, flanks, thighs, and neck.

BODY CONDITION SCORING

BCS 1 = emaciation: little muscle, no fat, concave contour.
  BCS 3 = good condition: convex contour, little subcutaneous fat.

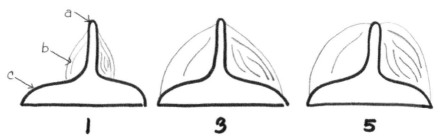

Fig. 2. Transverse sections of the sternum and pectoral muscle mass in the avian patient displaying body condition score (BCS) where (a) is the keel or carina of the sternum, (b) is pectoral musculature, and (c) is the sternum.[9] (Permission gained from Christal Pollock, DVM for image above – Reference #9 - Pollock C. Body condition scoring in birds. October, 2012. LafeberVet Web site. Available at https://lafeber.com/vet/body-condition-scoring/ Accessed April 30, 2023.)

BCS 5 = obese: contour extends beyond keel, subcutaneous fat deposits.

Fat is frequently deposited within subcutaneous tissues, especially over the coelom and lateral flanks, in birds that are overweight. It is important that the patient be physically examined and observed while standing, as subcutaneous fat deposits in the inguinal area may result in a broad-based stance in the overweight patient. Fat deposits underneath the beak can create the appearance of what is termed in humans as a "double chin." In addition, fat deposits along either side of the keel can also create a part in feathers overlying the sternum, often referred to as cleavage. The veterinary team should also be cognizant of the potential for lipomas in morbidly obese patients, particularly budgerigar budgerigars and Amazon parrots.[9]

BCS is useful as a cursory determination of emaciation. However, veterinary teams must remember that most companion birds do not store fat in their pectoral region and may have significant fat deposits while still having an apparently normal body score. To complete the evaluation of body condition it is recommended to wet the feathers over the abdomen, flanks, thighs, and neck with alcohol; this allows for visualization of subcutaneous fat deposits, which can be visually observed as yellow fat under the skin as opposed to pinkish-red muscle.[10] To obtain a complete and accurate assessment of body condition in avian patients, the combination of recording the current body weight, palpation and scoring of the pectoral muscle, and visual assessment of subcutaneous fat should all be performed.

It is important to remember that body condition cannot be assessed by palpation of the pectoral muscle mass in pediatric patients, as the pectoral muscle at this time is small, soft, and flabby.[9] As an alternative in pediatric patients, it is best to evaluate the amount of soft tissue and fat over bony areas such as the pelvis and toes.

AVIAN KEY NUTRITIONAL FACTORS
Energy

The definition of basal metabolic rate (BMR) is the amount of energy expended by a healthy bird under thermoneutral conditions, 12 hours after a meal, and the bird is at rest.[11,12] To calculate the BMR the following equation is used with a K value for psittacine birds of 175:

$$BMR = K\,(W_{kg})0.75 = kcal/day \; Or \; BMR = 175\,(W_{kg})0.75 = kcal/day.$$

Increase in energy expenditure over BMR (as reported in Budgies) is as follows:

Activity	Increase Over BMR
Perching	2x
Preening	2.3x
Eating	2.3x
Minor movement around cage	2.3x
Flight	11–20x

Free-living birds' energy requirements are higher than the requirements of captive birds because of the increased energy required for thermoregulation, food procurement, and territorial defense. Yet, the daily requirements for amino acids, minerals, and vitamins are constant despite the level of energy expenditure. Climate can influence BMR as seen in Psittacines from temperate climates that have BMRs approximately 20% higher than tropical Psittacine species.[11]

Energy derived from food is released from protein, carbohydrates, fats, and other organic compounds. Although not a chemically definable nutrient, energy is a property that nutrients possess. When the 3 key calorigenic nutrients (carbohydrates, fats, proteins) in a food are burnt entirely with enough oxygen, it releases energy or food calories that are expressed in kilojoules (kJ) or kilocalories (kcal). Food energy is usually measured by a bomb calorimeter based on the heat of combustion.[13]

Energy released by a particular food is a critical parameter in nutrition. Several chronic diseases such as obesity, diabetes, and cardiovascular disease are considered to be caused by excess energy intake.

The physiology of a particular avian species determines its nutrient requirements. Requirements are determined for 3 physiologic states: basal, maintenance, and total. The basal requirements are those needed to maintain basic life functions and keep the patient alive. The maintenance requirement is the amount of nutrients needed for basal functions, coupled with the activity of finding and consuming food, interacting with other animals, and maintaining body temperature. The total energy requirement is the combination of all requirements for life and its stages, including growth, reproduction, and molt.[6]

Water

Water is the most critical nutrient, and all birds should have access to fresh, clean water at all times. There are a few avian species that have evolved from arid regions (budgerigars) and can survive several months without drinking, apparently relying on water derived from metabolic sources. These few species are the exception, as most companion birds drink water daily. If water is not provided the bird will become distressed and may die within 48 hours. Water should be changed daily, and the health care team is responsible for reviewing this important piece of husbandry with owners. The consumption of water will increase in breeding birds with hatchlings in the nest or when the bird is subjected to warmer temperatures. Birds typically accept municipal tap water, but it is recommended that well water be boiled before allowing the bird to drink freely. If owners are hesitant to boil water, the health care team should recommend providing bottled water to their birds. This recommendation is made because of the fact that well water can be contaminated easily by bacteria colonies in the pipes leading to the faucet.[1–3,14]

Adding any compound to the drinking water may render the water unpalatable, thus reducing water consumption and increasing the potential for dehydration and death. This is particularly true in diseased birds. Adding medications to drinking water may be an inaccurate and potentially dangerous way of delivering medications. It is best for the veterinary team to avoid this method of medication administration. Supplementing vitamins and minerals using drinking water is also not recommended. Water intake can vary inter- and intraspecifically, and intake is influenced by diet and environmental temperatures. The high oxidation-reduction capabilities of minerals, (eg, zinc, iron, copper) may eliminate vitamins. In addition, some vitamins are light-sensitive. Attempting to standardize intake of vitamins via drinking water is impossible. In fact, it has been reported that vitamin A and D toxicoses have occurred in macaws and conures being supplemented with liquid vitamins.[11,15] Dehydration may result if the additives decrease water intake due to unpleasant taste or unfamiliar coloration.

Proper water and water dish husbandry should be reinforced with bird owners, as bacterial contamination of water or of foods with a high moisture content is also a health risk. Veterinary teams should educate owners that water containers should be regularly cleaned and disinfected and fresh, clean water provided at least once a day.

Protein and Amino Acids

Protein requirements differ among species. The levels of protein consumed must meet the nitrogen requirements for the particular avian species in its housing condition and life stage. Birds in a specific dietary strategy (eg, granivorous birds) that have an increased body size also have higher requirements of protein than smaller species.[6]

The largest portion of protein mass in birds is feathers. For example, feathers of budgerigars represent 5.7% of the protein mass, which accounts for 28% of the total body protein. Molt also requires increased protein needs.[6] Feathers are enriched with cysteine along with several nonessential amino acids. During a feather's formation, these amino acids are continually incorporated into the feather; this differs from gastrointestinal tract uptake, as this only occurs after consuming a meal, when amino acids are manufactured from sources of tissue protein. Energy is lost during molt because the bird loses insulation during the molt, thus requiring increased energy. In addition, there are increased expenditures to obtain more protein to synthesize feather proteins.[6]

As with all foods, the quality of the protein depends on bioavailability and essential amino acid content. Bird food formulations must avoid excess and deficiency of proteins and amino acids. For most of the companion birds the following amino acids are considered essential: arginine, isoleucine, lysine, methionine, phenylalanine, valine, tryptophan, and threonine. Budgies also require glycine.[2,14,16]

Too much protein in the diet of birds has been associated with renal disease, behavioral changes (biting, feather picking, nervousness, rejection of food), and regurgitation. Poor weight gain, poor feathering, stress lines on feathers, plumage color changes, and poor reproductive performance are clinical signs associated with protein and amino acid deficiencies.[16]

Fats and Essential Fatty Acids

Fats are a more concentrated source of energy in a diet. Essential fatty acids (linoleic and arachidonic) are required in birds for the following: the formation of membranes and cell organelles, hormone precursors, and the basis for psittacofulvins (ie, feather pigments found in psittacine species). The typical recommended fat allowance for granivorous companion bird diets is approximately 4%.[1,16] It is important for health care team members to note that in birds, lipogenesis takes place primarily in the liver. Pet birds fed high-energy diets may develop illness associated with hepatic lipidosis; this is heightened if exercise is restricted in the bird.

n-6 and n-3 polyunsaturated fatty acids (PUFAs) play a role in and can affect the following:

- Immunity and its response
- Cardiovascular system health
- Nervous system health
- Improves renal function
- Reduces osteoarthritis.

PUFAs affect immune function in 3 ways: (1) altering eicosanoid synthesis, (2) altering cell membranes that affect membrane-associated protein and receptor functions, and (3) modifying fatty acid pools that affect cytokine production. Overall, omega-3 fatty acids produce fewer inflammatory cytokines and are considered antiinflammatory. The omega-6 fatty acid, arachidonic acid, is the precursor for prostaglandins, leukotrienes, and other related compounds that produce proinflammatory cytokines. The antiinflammatory role of the n-3 fatty acids from marine fish oils (eicosapentaenoic acid and docosahexaenoic acid) have been found to have a beneficial effect in cardiovascular and inflammatory/autoimmune diseases.[6,17]

As with other companion animals and humans, too much fat in the diet of a bird may result in obesity, hepatic lipidosis, congestive heart failure, diarrhea, and oily feather texture. Increased fat levels may also interfere with the absorption of other nutrients such as calcium. Low amounts of fat in the diet may lead to weight loss, reduced disease resistance, and overall poor growth, especially when coupled with restriction of other energy-producing nutrients.[1,11]

Carbohydrates

Dietary carbohydrates aid in the production of energy in the form of adenosine triphosphate from glycolysis and the tricarboxylic acid cycle.[11] Carbohydrates play an important role in many processes in the body:

- Produce heat from the oxidation of glucose to CO_2 and H_2O
- Aid in production of precursors of other nutrients
- Synthesize glycogen or fat from glucose
- Decrease pH of the lumina through production of short-chain fatty acids
- Increase the number of anaerobic flora

The antibacterial properties of short-chain fatty acids aid in decreasing pathogenic intestinal bacteria. They also aid in the prevention of, and recovery from, intestinal disorders.

It is important to note that one of the predominant disaccharides of fruit sugars, sucrose, is readily digestible. In species that lack the sucrase enzyme, the differences in proportions of fruit mono- and disaccharides are important. It is recommended to avoid feeding these birds fruits high in disaccharides (eg, mango, apricot, nectarine, and so forth).

Carbohydrates are an energy source that in birds can be converted into fat in the liver and vice versa. Glucagon is the major component of carbohydrate metabolism in birds. The result of inadequate carbohydrates in the diet is the utilization of glucogenic amino acids to manufacture carbohydrates. The process involves amino acids being shifted away from growth and production and instead used in glucose synthesis.[2,11]

Carbohydrates are the only source of energy utilizable by the nervous system; therefore, neurological abnormalities may indicate deficiency in a diet that is otherwise adequate in kilojoule content.[1,11]

Calcium

Calcium is an important dietary element for companion pet birds. Calcium is essential for bone and eggshell formation. Calcium is also necessary for blood coagulation and nerve and muscle function.

It is recommended that all birds should have calcium supplementation in their cage regardless of the type of diet they are eating. This is especially true for birds fed a seed diet. Calcium supplementation can be provided in the form of a cuttlebone, mineral block, crushed oyster shell, or baked crushed eggshell. Birds will eat the calcium if provided and when needed to meet physiologic demands. Cuttlebones should be placed in the cage with the soft side facing the bird. Cuttlebones are strictly a calcium source and are not beak sharpening devices.[2,5] It should also be noted that high phosphorus in the diet can negate adequate amounts of calcium in the diet. High phosphorous levels will interfere with calcium absorption from the intestinal tract. The calcium to phosphorus ratio should be range from 1:1 to 2:1[5,11]; this is another reason to provide a nutritionally balanced diet, as seeds, fruit, vegetables, meat are extremely calcium-deficient but do have higher amounts of phosphorous. For example, corn has a 1:37 ratio, and muscle meat has a 1:20 ratio.[5]

VITAMINS AND MINERALS

Overall, vitamin requirements for companion birds are similar to those of companion mammals. However, there are a few vitamins that are discussed, as they relate to psittacines.

Vitamin A

The vitamin most likely to be deficient in the diets of both captive and wild birds is vitamin A due to the variability of vitamin A amounts consumed in the avian diet. Vitamin A signifies those noncarotenoid derivatives with biological activity comparable with trans-retinols. Most occur as retinol and retinol esters that are absorbed from the gastrointestinal tract and transported for storage in the liver.[6,18] Vitamin A has 2 cell functions: (1) the hormonelike regulatory actions of retinoic acid and (2) the photoreceptor actions of retinal. The exact requirement of vitamin A is unknown in psittacine birds. Vitamin A deficiency in psittacine birds manifests the following:

- Signs of keratinization of their mucous membranes
- Anorexia
- Poor conditioning
- Increased infection vulnerability

Parrots may exhibit salivary gland metaplasia, including their excretory ducts and glandular epithelium. Vitamin A status has also been shown to affect vocalizations in cockatiels.[18]

Deficiency of vitamin A also damages the function of the rods in the eyes and may lead to night blindness in birds. Although, if caught early, feeding adequate amounts of vitamin A can reverse this in just a few days.[19] Severe vitamin A deficiencies result in keratinization of the conjunctiva with insufficient corneal lubrication, thus leading to abrasions and potential sight loss.

Carotenoids in the diet serve as vitamin A precursors. Carotenoids such as beta-carotene can be degraded enzymatically in the intestinal epithelium; this helps to form retinal (one form of vitamin A) and can then be converted to other forms such as retinol and retinoic acid. The needs of the body aid in regulating the conversion of carotenoids to vitamin A. Because of this, consumption of beta-carotenoids is a safe alternative versus feeding vitamin A directly.[19]

Vitamin C

Vitamin C is involved in many physiologic processes such as the syntheses of collagen, carnitine, and catecholamine, the metabolism of fatty acids and medications, and in peroxidation prevention. Stressed birds, including the stresses associated with high temperatures, growth, and reproduction, may have increased requirements for vitamin C.

Most avian patients synthesize vitamin C in the kidney, liver, or both. Fresh fruits, green leafy vegetables, and animal organs have higher concentrations of vitamin C, with only small amounts in skeletal muscle. Improper handling and processing can destroy vitamin C. When exposed to boiling water for short periods of time vitamin C remains stable. A greater percentage is destroyed when subjected to heat at low temperatures for longer periods. Freezing and thawing or any type of processing that ruptures tissue subjects vitamin C to air losses due to oxidation. Vitamin C has been found to be stable during normal pelleting processes.[11]

Vitamin C is important in specific fruit-eating species, but for most of the psittacine species a complete and balanced diet will provide the necessary amounts of vitamin C. However, vitamin C supplementation has been suggested to assist debilitated birds, as the ability to create vitamin C is reduced and the patients' requirements are greater.[1,11]

Vitamin D

The activity of vitamin D is observed in a group of related sterols including cholecalciferol (vitamin D3), ergosterol (vitamin D2), and other metabolites. Birds can synthesize cholecalciferol in their skin from cholesterol; however, this requires an adequate amount of sunlight to do so. Most companion birds do not have adequate ultraviolet exposure for endogenous conversion; thus, they need to attain vitamin D through a dietary source. Overall, birds do not have the ability to convert ergosterol (the form available for cats and dogs) into cholecalciferol for use in metabolism.[1,2] Instead, this form of vitamin D is excreted in the bile. If birds are able to receive adequate sunlight, they do not have a specific requirement for vitamin D3. Vitamin D toxicity results in increased mobilization of calcium with soft tissue mineralization including joints, kidneys, myocardium, blood vessels, and the pancreas. Tubule calcification in the kidney may lead to a fatal buildup of excretory products.

Vitamin E

There are 2 groups of compounds with antioxidant activity that make up vitamin E—the alpha-tocopherols and the gamma-tocotrienols. The most biologically active form of vitamin E is the D-tocopherol, which is used as the dietary standard. Only the alpha-tocopherols are incorporated into the tissues of birds. Plasma lipoproteins transport vitamin E, which is then incorporated into the lipid bilayer of the cell's membranes. Vitamin E stabilizes these membranes and quenches reactions of oxygen intermediates and polyunsaturated fatty acids. Alpha-tocopherols compete for free radicals and work synergistically with several enzymes (superoxide dismutase, glutathione peroxidase, and catalase) to protect cell membranes. To function properly, these enzymes require trace minerals as cofactors, including zinc, manganese, selenium, and iron. If these are found to be deficient, the absolute requirement of vitamin E increases, and this further shows that many of the nutrients are linked.

The levels of vitamin E required in the diet vary, depending on several factors:

- Levels of polyunsaturated fatty acids,
- Levels of vitamin A and/or beta-carotene,
- Presence and quantity of other dietary antioxidants,
- Rancidity of fats in the diet, and
- The content of selenium.

Selenium deficiencies can lead to an impairment of the glutathione peroxidase antioxidant system, thus increasing the need for vitamin E.

Vitamin E deficiencies manifest as symptoms related to cell membrane dysfunction. Commonly observed symptoms include encephalomalacia, exudative diathesis, muscular dystrophy, myopathy of the ventriculus, and increased fragility of red blood cells.

Vitamin E is synthesized by plants, and alpha-tocopherols are mainly found in plant leaves. Gamma tocopherols are found more regularly in vegetable oils and grains. In birds, the most active form of vitamin E is alpha-tocopherol. Foods high in vitamin E include green leafy vegetables, egg yolks, palm nuts, and canola oil.

If the bird is prescribed antibiotics, the health care team should monitor the patient closely, as vitamin deficiencies may result from the antibiotics interfering with normal intestinal microflora. Intestinal infections (eg, giardiasis) may block vitamin absorption from the intestine (eg, vitamin E, vitamin A). Hypervitaminosis has become an increasing problem, as clients may oversupplement formulated food or multivitamin preparations, thereby causing renal failure due to hypervitaminosis D. Hypervitaminosis A can also result in disease, especially in nectarivorous (those birds that eat the sugar-rich nectar of flowering plants or the juices of fruits) birds.[1,2,11]

Vitamin K

Vitamin K is responsible for revealing antihemorrhagic activity. Vitamin K functions as a cofactor of a hepatic microsomal carboxylase. Carboxylation is necessary for the function of proteins including osteocalcin; clotting factors VII, IX, and X; and prothrombin.[6] Compared with other fat-soluble vitamins, vitamin K experiences rapid turnover in tissues and is not stored for periods of time in the liver. Although the requirement of vitamin K in the body is low, it is essential for the clotting mechanism. In addition, requirements increase with infection and with the presence of vitamin K antagonists. These antagonists include dicumarols produced by molds from grains. Another antagonist is long-term antibiotic administration, which reduces normal intestinal microflora. Psittacines with liver failure that eat seed-only diets have had uncontrolled hemorrhage, usually resulting from a broken blood feather in a hospital setting.

Typically, vitamin K is supplemented with a water-soluble form of menadione to alleviate potential toxicity. Leaves of plants are rich sources of vitamin K, whereas fruits, soybean meal, and seeds are poor sources.[19]

FRUITS AND VEGETABLES

Fruits and vegetables are typically presented as supplementation to the pet birds' commercial diet. Fruits are made up of mainly sugars and water and thus should not be offered in excess. Fruit is a necessary part of the diet for some psittacine species such as eclectus and lories, but these are exceptions. Fruit should not be fed more than a couple of times in a 7-day period.

Companion birds receive greater nutritional benefit from vegetables as opposed to fruits. As much as possible, fresh or cooked dark green, red, and orange vegetables should be offered on a daily basis. One vegetable that should NOT be offered is comfrey. Comfrey is a green leaf herb especially popular in canary aviaries, which may lead to liver damage. Proper husbandry suggests the health care team educate owners to place fruit and vegetables in a separate container and leave it in cage no longer than 30 minutes. Time restriction will help decrease the likelihood of microorganism growth.[2,5]

DIET FORMULATION

It is suggested that a balanced diet be provided, and to best achieve a balanced diet, a formulated food should be fed. These formulated foods come in a variety of forms with the most popular being[2,6]:

1. Pellets
2. Extruded diets with a pellet appearance
3. Whole grains and/or seeds with added pelleted material

A seed-based food with a vitamin/mineral mix coating on the outside of the seed is another option. However, most often the seed is not hulled. When the bird dehulls the coated seed, necessary vitamins and minerals are removed, thus creating a nutritional imbalance putting the bird's health at risk.

Two processes are used when pelleted diets are manufactured—bound and extruded. Bound pellet manufacturing involves the grinding of grains such as corn, soybean, and oat groats (oat berries). Following the grinding process vitamins, minerals, and other components are added to produce a balanced food (per the manufacturer's recommendation). The grinding process produces a consistent pellet, which makes it difficult for birds to pick out their favorite part of the diet. With bound pellets in general, the food material is not cooked, and the diet will have a longer fiber chain length. Bound pelleted diets may not be as palatable as the extruded diet.[2,5,6]

Extruded pellets use finely ground grains that are mixed with vitamins, minerals, and so forth until a balanced formulation is reached. This pellet mixture is then forced through an extruder, under pressure and high temperatures. The mixture will take on the shape of the "die" in the extrusion process; this allows for extruded pellets to be made into different shapes and colours.[5,6]

Extruded pelleted diets come in a variety of sizes and should be selected based on the species and size of bird. Owners must be instructed to monitor their bird to prevent picking out certain colored pellets and ignoring others. Owners should not choose colors or shapes because their bird "likes these," as this can be expensive and wasteful. Companion birds are healthier when they are psychologically stimulated, and this can occur by presenting multicolored pellets in an assortment of shapes.[2] Historically, providing diets for birds has included seed-based diets. Although pelleted diets have allowed bird owners to provide a better balanced diet without vitamin and mineral supplementation, not every bird will eat them.[2] Also as discussed earlier, each species has different nutritional requirements. For the psittacine species seed is not the recommended diet, and a balanced pelleted food is advised as the appropriate base diet. Overall, many seed diets are high in fat and lower in other essential nutrients and therefore should be considered a treat. As with any species, treats should be offered in small quantities, or the bird will be at risk of obesity.

Transition from a seed diet to a pellet is believed to be difficult. However, this is not the case even in older birds. Health care team members must educate owners on what to look for when transitioning a bird from seed to pellets. Owners should ensure that their pet is ingesting the food, not simply crushing the pellet in the hopes of finding a kernel inside. Two signs that indicate that the bird is actually eating the pellets are seen in the production of fecal material and a color change of the fecal material associated with the pellet color being ingested.[2,5]

To aid owners in transitioning their birds from seed to pellet, formed seed products have been manufactured (ie, Nutriberries Lafeber Co., Cornell, IL, USA). These products are composed of whole grains and seeds that are mixed with additional components and are stuck together; this is similar to pellets, but this product is not ground. The bird must pick off the seed to eat.

Owners can also learn to transition their birds from seed to pellets through the slow introduction of increased pellets in the seed mixture over a period of time. The transition is recommended to take 7 to 14 days, with the final diet consisting of 100% pellets.

OBESITY

Wild birds spend most of their day forging for food, often flying (sometimes miles) to find a proper feeding ground. When they have located an area in which to feed, they are often climbing up and down trees and flying to other trees or other areas. Sadly, the sedentary lifestyle of the companion bird often results in obesity, which is one of the most common forms of malnutrition presenting to veterinary hospitals.

As in other taxonomic groups, obesity is a disease that puts pet birds at risk for potential disease conditions (eg, cardiovascular disease, diabetes mellitus, liver disease, respiratory disease, neoplasia), as well as increase mortality risk. One study in canines found that dogs fed ad libitum are more prone to be overweight, thus resulting in a shortened lifespan.[20] A wealth of information is now available to demonstrate the adverse health effects that can arise when any pet becomes overweight. In pet birds, hyperadiposity increases the risk of developing.

- Lipomas
- Xanthomatosis
- Osteoarthritis
- Hepatic lipidosis
- Diabetes mellitus
- Renal disease
- Herniation
- Cardiovascular disease
- Respiratory compromise (air sac compression)
- Hypertension
- Atherosclerosis
- Egg binding
- Dystocia
- Cloacal prolapse
- Infertility

Diets with excess energy content contribute to weight gain and increase the risk of developing these disease conditions. In addition, excess fat may limit the absorption of calcium.[21] Inactivity, specifically lack of flight, has been listed as the main cause of developing the aforementioned medical issues in captive parrots. In addition, high-energy diets have also been linked to the development of these issues in captive and inactive birds. Medium- and large-sized parrots are more likely to develop atherosclerosis than smaller psittacine species (pers. obs.). Frugivorous species are also more prone to obesity and hepatic lipidosis if their low protein and energy requirements are exceeded.[22] Behavioral problems such as depression, repetitive movements, and feather destructive behavior can also be seen in sedentary birds.

There are several potential causes of obesity in birds. Most prominent are consumption of high-fat diets, excess caloric intake, insufficient exercise, and species predisposition. Just as in other species—too much energy in and too little energy expended.

Companion bird species that seem to be at higher risk for obesity include Amazon parrots (*Amazona* spp), Budgerigar parakeets (*Melopsittacus undulates*), cockatiels (*Nymphicus hollandicus*), and cockatoos, as well as quaker or monk parakeets (*Myiopsitta monachus*).[22,23]

Body weight relative to a bird's optimal weight has been used as a defining criterion for obesity because body weight is easier to measure than body fat. Body weight in excess of optimal body weight of 1% to 9% is acceptable, 10% to 19% is considered overweight, and greater than 20% is defined as obese.[11]

OBESITY PREVENTION

It is imperative that the veterinary team recognize that obesity is a disease state. Adipose tissue is no longer considered to be solely a depot for energy. Rather adipose tissue actively produces hormones involved in energy homeostasis in addition to cytokines, recognized as important modulators of inflammation. Obesity is a state of chronic, low-grade inflammation.[24]

In addition, it is imperative that the veterinary team perform a physical examination, history, and nutritional history to accurately determine the patient's health status, any testing that may be necessary, body weight, BCS, what the bird is eating, how much it is eating, and what exercise the patient is receiving. This information aids the team in tailoring the weight loss program to the individual patient.

It is clear that weight management relies on reduction of caloric intake while increasing exercise. However, it is also understood that most weight loss programs will fail without proper client communication and education.[25] To this end, the bird owner must agree to the following:

- Understand and agree their bird is overweight
- Understand the need for the weight loss recommendation
- Is willing and able to work with the team to address the problem.

If high calorie and high-energy food items are noted (seeds, nuts, some fruits), work with the owner to gradually reduce these items while gradually increasing lower calorie items, such as vegetables. The introduction of a formulated diet and education of how this diet benefits the avian patient can also reduce confusion and subjectivity associated with many pet bird diets. Formulated therapeutic diets low in energy and fat and high in fiber (ie, Lafeber's Nutri-An Cakes for Foraging and Weight Maintenance) can also prove helpful.

It is critical to discuss how much of the recommended food to feed, and include any vegetables, fruits, treats, and so forth, in the calculation and owner discussion. Write this recommendation down for the owner and in the medical record. Ensure owner understanding before discharge and have them repeat the instructions back to the team member.

Encourage the owner to provide the bird with enrichment and foraging opportunities. Enrichment involves providing an environment that allows the bird to express natural behaviors in a captive or caged condition.[23] Encourage foraging behavior with the bird's food. By linking foraging foods with objects and toys, the birds' captive behaviors are heightened, and the brain is stimulated. Foraging is a natural behavior; therefore, to satisfy this behavior, birds in home environments need to learn to forage in their cages to acquire their food.[23] Encourage foraging behavior with food-motivated play such as feeder puzzles and other enrichment tools. Also, discuss with owners the idea of increasing the size of the cage to add a variety of perches, toys, swings, ladders, and multiple perch play gyms to allow for increased activity.

Ensure a proper health screening before recommending a weight loss program. The veterinary team should be sure to manage and stabilize any problems identified before the implementation of an exercise regimen. Discuss expectations that may result from the enrichment program, such as some birds will begin gradual wing flapping.[23] This is a positive response to interactive play exercise.

When implementing a weight loss program, it is important to involve all members of the household; this aids in ensuring all family members understand the weight loss program and how it affects the health of their bird. Understanding and acceptance leads to compliance, and compliance leads to better health for the patient. Remember to provide clear, concise, and simple instructions. It has been shown that clients remember information given during the first third of any communication. Given this, it is important for the veterinary team to organize the information provided appropriately.

Follow-up is crucial to success. Follow-up allows the team to monitor patient progress and adjust the weight loss program as needed. It also allows for client support. Weight management programs in any species can be difficult. Troubleshooting, communicating, and supporting the bird owner help to keep the weight loss program on track. Have the owner use the same scale and weigh the bird at the same time of day. Encourage them to track their birds' progress and initially schedule follow-up visits at 1- to 2-week intervals. Follow-up calls should be done sooner.

Once the bird has reached its optimal body weight, celebrate with the owner. Remind them that recheck examinations are still needed. Maintaining this ideal weight can be difficult, especially given that it is natural to revert to former habits.

SUMMARY

Nutrition is the one factor that the veterinary health care team can affect. Proper nutrition and feeding management are the foundation of good health. Optimal feeding practices of companion birds are constantly being evaluated. It is critical that health care team members understand the key nutritional factors in avian nutrition, as this allows for the proper recommendation and education of nutrition to bird owners. Pet bird owners influence their bird's diet and therefore have a major impact on their bird's health and longevity. Depending on the species, today's pet birds may live decades, so it is imperative that proper nutrition habits be adopted by the owner for their avian pet. Educating the owner on proper nutrition and prevention of obesity is one of the most important roles of the veterinary health care team.

CLINICS CARE POINTS

- Psittacines have specific nutritional requirements, determined by individual physiology.
- The veterinary health care team should recognize that nutritional deficiencies or imbalances resulting from primary or secondary disease are common.

- Every bird that presents to the hospital, every time they present, should be assessed to establish nutritional needs and feeding goals.
- Obesity in pet birds is becoming much more common.

DISCLOSURE

The author does consult with the Lafeber Company.

REFERENCES

1. Macwhirter P. Basic anatomy, physiology, and nutrition. In: Tully TN, Dorrestein GM, Jones AK, editors. Handbook of avian medicine. 2nd ed. St. Louis: Elsevier; 2009. p. 24–54.
2. Burns KM. Avian nutrition: it's for the birds. Today's Veterinary Nurse. Fall; 2021. p. 14–7.
3. Burns KM. Avian nutrition. In: Wortinger A, Burns KM, editors. Nutrition and disease management for veterinary technicians and nurses. 2nd edition. Ames (IA): Wiley Blackwell; 2015. p. 227–33.
4. Harcourt-Brown NH. Psittacine birds. In: Tully TN, Dorrestein GM, Jones AK, editors. Handbook of avian medicine. 2nd ed. St. Louis: Elsevier; 2009. p. 137–67.
5. Tully T. Birds. In: Mitchell M, Tully T, editors. Manual of exotic pet practice. St. Louis: Saunders Elsevier; 2009. p. 250–98.
6. Orosz S. Clinical avian nutrition. Vet Clin Exot Anim 2014;17:397–413.
7. Cline M, Burns KM, Coe JB, et al. AAHA nutrition and weight management guidelines for dogs and cats. J Am Anim Hosp Assoc 2021;57(4):153–78.
8. Burns KM. Implementing a nutritional assessment for your feline patients. Spring: The Feline Practitioner; 2023. p. 44–8.
9. Pollock C. Body condition scoring in birds. October, 2012. LafeberVet Web site. Available at: https://lafeber.com/vet/body-condition-scoring/. Accessed April 30, 2023.
10. Doneley B, Harrison GJ, Lightfoot TL. Maximizing information from the physical examination. In: Harrison GJ, Lightfoot TL, editors. Clinical avian medicine. vols. 1 & 2. Spix Publishing, Inc. Palm Beach, FL 2005. p. 153–212.
11. McDonald D. Nutrition and dietary supplementation. In: Harrison GJ, Lightfoot TL, editors. Clinical avian medicine. vols. 1 & 2. Spix Publishing, Inc. Palm Beach, FL. 2005. p. 86–107.
12. Pollock C. Estimating energy requirements. January 13, 2013. LafeberVet Web site. Available at: https://lafeber.com/vet/estimating-energy-requirements/. Accessed May 2, 2023.
13. Jiang B, Tsao R, Li Y, et al. Food safety: food analysis technologies/techniques. In: Van Alfen Neal K, editor. Encyclopedia of Agriculture and Food Systems. San Diego (CA): Academic Press; 2014. p. 273–88.
14. Burns KM. Nutrition for companion birds. The RVT Journal 2014;37(4):6–9.
15. Schoemaker NJ, Lumeij JT, Beynen AC. Polyuria and polydipsia due to vitamin and mineral oversupplementation of the diet of a salmon crested cockatoo (*Cacatua moluccensis*) and a blue and gold macaw (*Ara ararauna*). Avian Pathol 1997;26:201–9.
16. Brue RN. Nutrition. In: Ritchie B, Harrison G, Harrison L, editors. Avian medicine: principles and application. Lake Worth, FL: Wingers; 1994. p. 70–85.

17. Anderson M, Fritsche KL. (n-3) Fatty acids and infectious disease resistance. J Nutr 2002;132:3566–76.
18. Koutsos EA, Matson KD, Klasing KC. Nutrition of birds in the order Psittaciformes: a review. J Avian Med Surg 2001;15:257–75.
19. Klasing KC. Vitamins. In: Klasing KC, editor. Comparative avian nutrition. New York: CABI Publishing; 1998. p. 277–329.
20. Kealy RD, Lawler DF, Ballam JM, et al. Effects of diet restriction on life span and age-related changes in dogs. J Am Vet Med Assoc 2002;220:1315–20.
21. Harper EJ, Skinner ND. Clinical nutrition of small psittacines and passerines. Seminars Avian Exot Pet Med 1998;7:116–27.
22. Perpinan D. Problems of excess nutrients in psittacine diets. Companion animal 2015;20(9):2–7.
23. Pollock C. Nutritional management of obesity in birds. October 1, 2012. Lafeber-Vet Web site. Available at: https://lafeber.com/vet/obesity/. Accessed April 30, 2023.
24. Michel KE. Nutritional management of body weight. In: Fascetti AJ, Delaney SJ, editors. Applied veterinary clinical nutrition. Ames, Iowa: Wiley-Blackwell; 2012. p. 109–24.
25. Burns K. Helping an Overweight Dog Lose Weight. Veterinary Team Brief/Clinician's Brief. November/December 2018, 42–5.

An Update on Key Nutritional Factors in Ferret Nutrition

Cayla Iske, PhD

KEYWORDS

- Ferret • Nutrition • Diet • Carnivore • Pet

KEY POINTS

- Ferrets should be exposed to a combination of canned, extruded, freeze-dried/fresh, and whole prey foods.
- Fat concentrations in the diet should be considered as heavily as protein, with a targeted protein-to-fat ratio of 2:1.
- Plant-derived ingredients, particularly plant-based proteins, are not well utilized by ferrets and could have health consequences.
- Concentrations and ratios of minerals should be considered and deserve further evaluation in ferret diets.

INTRODUCTION

The modern-day pet ferret belongs to the mustelid family of carnivorous mammals, joined by mink, weasels, and badgers. Not to be confused with the black-footed ferret (*Mustela nigripes*), the domestic ferret (*Mustela putorius furo*) has been domesticated for over 2000 years.[1] Though their original use and purpose was related to hunting, and in some cases fur production, today millions of ferrets are owned as pets and in the early 2000s ferrets were considered the third most popular pet.[2] In recent years, ferrets have also become a popular model for human biomedical research including respiratory diseases, virology, and gastrointestinal diseases.[3] Popularity as pets and use in lab animal research have led to a focus on care and husbandry over the past decade. A large part of that has been emphasis on improved nutrition.

Anatomy and Physiology

The in-depth anatomy of ferrets has been described by previous authors.[4] Highlights specific to nutrition include an extremely short digestive tract and transit time, no cecum, simple stomach and microflora, and limited brush border enzymes.[5–7] It has also been described that ferrets spontaneously secrete hydrochloric acid.[6,7] Perhaps,

Omaha's Henry Doorly Zoo & Aquarium, 3701 South 10th Street, Omaha, NE 68107, USA
E-mail address: cayla.beebe-iske@omahazoo.com

Vet Clin Exot Anim 27 (2024) 31–45
https://doi.org/10.1016/j.cvex.2023.07.002
1094-9194/24/© 2023 Elsevier Inc. All rights reserved.

one of the most visually telling indicators of the natural diet of this species is the ferrets dentition and facial musculature. The large carnassial teeth and powerful bite force of the ferret indicate sheering and crushing are important feeding tactics.[7,8] All of these characteristics taken together point toward a diet nearly entirely composed of animal tissue, earning them the title of obligate carnivore.

The physiology of ferrets indicates small, frequent meals are part of their natural feeding style. Lack of cecum, limited brush border enzymes, and unsophisticated gut microflora describe an animal that consumes a diet low in carbohydrates of any kind, simple or complex. The length of the digestive tract cannot be overlooked. Relative to body length, ferret's small intestine is half as long as other carnivores, such as cats.[6] This is perhaps the most straightforward characteristic to shed light on important factors of ferret nutrition. With consumed food only spending approximately 3 hours in the gastrointestinal tract, it must be highly digestible. For ferrets, that means high in protein and fat and low in carbohydrates. Less apparent but equally as important when considering feeding ferrets, is the importance of the olfactory system. Smell is the sense that ferrets rely on the most, hence why they were originally used for hunting, and this develops very early in a ferret's life.[9]

Cats and mink have most commonly been used as models for the basis of ferret nutrition. While these models largely seem to suffice, there have been differences distinguished between these species. Cats were shown to have higher average digestibility values across nutrients and energy, and ferrets and mink seem to be more closely correlated than cats and ferrets.[10] However, ferrets did more efficiently digest fat compared to mink, indicating importance in the diet. Ferrets and mink also digested carbohydrates much less efficiently compared to cats, further emphasizing the hypercarnivorous diet of these species.[10] Diet of the wild ferret can also serve as a useful model when considering nutrition of the pet ferret.

Wild Diet Considerations

When formulating diets for human-managed exotic species, it is valuable to assess the diet of their wild counterparts. The nutrient composition of prey these animals consume in the wild can serve as a starting point for commercial formulations. When assessing remains in the digestive tracts or scat of wild ferrets in New Zealand, ferrets were found to consume a wide variety of species including rabbits, birds, opossums, hedgehogs, eggs, invertebrates, and reptiles, with seasonal variation.[11,12] Both of these studies found that rabbits constituted the majority of the diet for studied ferrets, accounting for 77% to 87% of prey consumed. Female ferrets were found to consume smaller prey items,[11] and also ate more non-rabbit prey items including more birds and invertebrates.[12] Birds and invertebrates were the second and third most commonly consumed prey items, comprising an average of 12.4% and 11.3%, respectively.[12] In a human-managed setting, ferrets are commonly offered mice, however, studies of wild ferrets show mice make up a small proportion of the diet at less than 5%.[11,12]

Though not perfect, extrapolating nutrient composition from whole prey fed in zoos can provide insight into the nutrient composition of wild ferret diets. Thus, published nutrient composition of rabbits, mice, and chickens can then be used as a tool to shed light on nutrient requirements of pet ferrets (**Table 1**).[13] From these analyses, it is clear that the diet of wild ferrets is high in moisture, protein, and fat. Data collected by this author suggest rabbits, adult mice, and chickens contain 2.2%, 1.1%, and 2.2% total dietary fiber on a dry matter basis (DMB), respectively. By calculation, nitrogen-free extract (NFE; simple carbohydrates) in these three prey species is 3.6% in rabbits, 8.1% in mice, and 3.2% in chickens (DMB). While fiber laboratory assays likely do not appropriately account for animal fiber (hair, skin, bones), potentially leading

Table 1 Nutrient composition of selected whole prey items on a dry matter basis[13]			
	Rabbit	Mouse	Chicken
Moisture, %	72.9	73.2	69.7
Crude Protein, %	67.3	57.9	55.0
Crude Fat, %	15.1	22.2	32.0
Ash, %	11.8	10.7	7.6
Nitrogen-Free Extract, %	3.6	8.1	3.2
Gross Energy, kcal/g	5.2	5.6	6.0
Calcium, %	2.6	2.7	1.8
Phosphorus, %	1.7	1.8	1.3
Magnesium, %	0.2	0.1	0.2
Sodium, %	0.4	0.4	0.6
Potassium, %	0.8	1.1	0.7
Copper, mg/kg	17.4	11.7	4.1
Iron, mg/kg	143.9	204.8	105.6
Zinc, mg/kg	74.9	91.3	78.8
Manganese, mg/kg	5.2	8.0	3.4
Vitamin A, IU/kg	6200	158,339	35,600
Vitamin E, IU/kg	38.1	68.0	51.3

to compound error in NFE calculations, these values suggest ferrets do not naturally consume or rely on carbohydrates in the diet. Furthermore, any simple carbohydrates in the diet come from the gut contents of prey animals.[9]

FEEDING THE PET FERRET

Using anatomy, physiology, and wild feeding habits of ferrets can guide best practices for pet ferret care and husbandry. Ferrets will eat up to 10 meals each day if given the choice and consume about 43 g of food per kilogram of body weight.[7,14] For this reason, many commercially available ferret foods recommend ad libitum feeding, which works well for most ferrets as they will self-regulate intake.[6] It should also be noted that seasonal fluctuations in weight and diet intake appear to be normal in wild and pet ferrets.[7,11,12] It has been documented that ferrets may consume up to 30% to 40% more food in the winter and gain a significant amount of weight.[6,7] This does not appear to be concerning as the weight will be shed in the spring by reducing food intake and metabolizing body fat. Monitoring of each individual's seasonal weight patterns can ensure regularity over the course of their lifetime.

Nutrient recommendations

Without a great deal of ferret-specific research to identify exact nutrient requirements, extrapolations from cats and mink are still largely used.[5,9] However, more research is being looked at specifically in ferrets to guide nutritional recommendations and formulations.

Protein
As ferrets are obligate carnivores, protein is the first focus of the diet. Published protein requirements for mink are 32.6% to 45.7% (DMB) for growing, gestating, or lactating animals and 21.8% to 26.0% at maintenance.[15] Dietary protein concentration of

30% to 40% crude protein (DMB) is often recommended for pet ferrets with no less than 35% protein recommended for gestating and lactating animals.[6,7,9,16] The particularly high protein requirement of ferrets could be due to digestive inefficiencies associated with a short digestive tract and/or related to first limiting amino acids.[5,9] Methionine is typically the first limiting amino acid in other carnivores-fed commercial diets, such as cats, largely due to available ingredients.[5] This is likely also the case for ferrets and has been highlighted in mink where a diet with as little as 28% protein, when supplemented with 0.6% methionine, showed the most growth and nitrogen balance compared with a higher protein (36%) diet.[17] Arginine is also an amino acid of focus as ferrets consuming diets containing below 0.4% arginine were shown to develop higer rates of hyperammonemia.[18] In addition to conjugation of bile acids, dietary taurine serves to conjugate xenobioitic acids in the ferret as well.[19] Additionally, the documentation of dilated cardiomyopathy (DMC) in pet ferrets and the link between DMC and taurine in cats cannot be ignored.[7,20] Though taurine deficiency has not been characterized in ferrets, most commercial feeds include it at a rate of approximately 0.25%.[5]

Fat

Dietary fat is an extremely important consideration in ferret nutrition, though often less talked about compared to protein. Fat in the diet should constitute the main source of calories.[6,7] Because fat contains twice as many calories as protein and carbohydrates,[21] due to its hydrophobic nature, the ratio of protein to fat can be targeted at approximately 2:1. Commercial diets with 20% to 25% fat have been well accepted and support healthy ferrets. Fat concentrations should be considered and weighed equally with protein when evaluating commercial ferret diets. Appropriate levels of fat, and specifically fatty acids, help with fat-soluble vitamin absorption as well as healthy skin and coat.[5,6] Ferrets are thought to require 3 essential fatty acids (EFA) for optimal growth and health: linoleic, linolenic, and arachidonic acid. The specific requirements for these fatty acids are not well defined, but for mink the total EFA concentrations of 0.5% (DMB) for maintenance and 1.5% for growing, pregnant, and lactating animals are recommended.[15] It is not uncommon for linoleic and linolenic acid (omega 6 and omega 3) to be declared on commercially available ferret foods, however, arachidonic acid is rarely stated. With a high-quality, meat-based diet, sufficient levels of arachidonic acid are usually present. Ratio of linoleic to linolenic acid is important due to the proinflammatory nature of a diet high in omega 6 fatty acids and anti-inflammatory nature of omega 3 fatty acids.[22] Though an ideal ratio for most species has not been scientifically determined, generally omega 6:omega 3 ratios of 2 to 10:1 should be targeted. Perhaps, one of the most practically important aspects of dietary fat in ferret diets is palatability. Palatability of ferret diets seems to be closely linked with fat concentrations, presentation, and source. Coating of kibble in animal fat tends to increase acceptance and palatability, with chicken fat seeming to be the preferred source.[6,7]

Energy

When evaluating the energy density of ferret diets, metabolizable energy (ME) rather than gross energy should be considered as it accounts only for the calories utilized by the animal.[5] Ferret diets containing around 4 kilocalories (kcals) per gram of food dry matter (DM) appear to support animals at every life stage.[5–7] Daily ME intakes for healthy ferrets at maintenance are estimated to be 200 to 300 kcals/kg of body weight.[5,7,9] So a 1.2 kg ferret would consume 240 to 360 kcals/d. On a diet with a caloric density of 4 kcal/g, this animal would consume 60 to 90 g of food each day. Daily energy requirements of growing, gestating, and lactating jills can triple from maintenance.[9]

Carbohydrates

Presumably, the only carbohydrates in the diet of a wild ferret come from the gut contents of their prey.[6,9] Physiologically, ferrets are not designed to digest and utilize carbohydrates. Growing ferrets fed a diet containing 27% protein, 17% fat, and 42% carbohydrates stopped growing and developed health issues, but these effects were not seen when the same animals were fed a diet composed of 38% protein, 18% fat, and 24% carbohydrates.[6] Commercially available ferret foods typically include binding agents for manufacturing (extrusion or pelleting) purposes as well as cost savings. These binding agents commonly come in the form of carbohydrate-rich ingredients such as wheat, oats, corn, or other grains. Though egg ingredients do serve as a binder, they are often cost prohibitive in formulation. Low levels of carbohydrates are hard to avoid in available ferret foods and though guaranteed analyses (GA) should show less than 3% to 5% crude fiber, total carbohydrate levels are higher. Carbohydrates can be calculated in the form of NFE if the food states moisture, protein, fat, fiber, and ash concentrations on the GA or if the food is analyzed for these components using the following equation: NFE = 100- (% Crude Protein + % Crude Fat + % Crude Fiber + % Moisture + % Ash).[23] Diets on the market today usually contain 20% to 30% carbohydrates, which are well tolerated by ferrets, though lower may be better.[5]

Water

Intake of dry food may be limited by the availability or intake of water, especially for young and gestating ferrets. It has been estimated that water intake of 60 mL/kg body weight daily is sufficient to support ferrets.[6,7,9] To encourage water consumption, multiple sources of water are recommended including multiple nontippable bowls in addition to a water bottle. Because ferrets are naturally playful and inquisitive, they love to play in water and will do so regularly. It is important to keep water sources clean and full, so fresh clean water is always available.

Vitamins and minerals

Mink and cats are used as appropriate models for most vitamin requirements of ferrets as little research has been conducted on ferret specifcally.[6,7] Previous authors have described dietary vitamin and mineral concentrations that appear to support ferrets and prevent deficiencies,[5–7] so this review will focus on key areas of focus and new research. Vitamin A is one nutrient for which models of ferret requirements deviate. Ferrets have been shown to absorb and store beta carotene and metabolize vitamin A more similarly to dogs than cats and rats.[24] Thus, ferret foods should be formulated using vitamin A requirements of dogs, 5000 IU/kg DM.[25] Vitamin sources in commercial products must withstand the heat of manufacturing and meet claimed GA values throughout shelf-life, typically 18 to 24 months. For this reason, commercial ferret foods commonly contain 25,000 to 37,000 IU/kg diet.[5] These diets are safe and support ferret health but safe upper limits of vitamin A for dogs (213,300 IU/kg DM) should not be exceeded.[25]

Vitamin E should be considered especially with diets high in polyunsaturated fatty acids (PUFA), such as fish-based or high fish inclusion diets. An alpha tocopherol to PUFA ratio of 0.6:1 (mg:g) has been recommended in humans and adopted for fox and mink diets to prevent oxidation.[15] Typically dietary concentrations of 185 to 250 IU/kg diet (assuming 60–90 g daily food intake this would be 7.4–15 mg vitamin E intake/d) support maintenance and growth but extremely high PUFA diets (>7.7% DMB) may require more vitamin E in the range of 75 to 150 mg daily (roughly 1250–3500 IU/kg diet) to prevent steatitis.[5,26] However, these high-PUFA, fish-based diets were fed to ferrets farmed for their coats and are not recommended for pet ferrets.[26]

The necessity of dietary vitamin K in ferrets is not established but germ-free ferrets did require vitamin K supplementation, suggesting it may be beneficial to healthy gut flora and microbiome.[27] Dry diets containing 1.0 mg menadione/kg food, and possibly less, support healthy plasma thrombin levels.[5] Currently, the only vitamin K supplement approved for use in pet food in the United States is menadione sodium bisulfite complex; no natural vitamin K supplement may legally be used.[23] This has led to some debate over its use and inclusion, however, currently dietary vitamin K supplementation is suggested.

Research regarding ideal dietary mineral concentrations is severely lacking in ferrets. However, most commercial foods, including many cat diets, appear to be adequate in minimum mineral concentrations. Fox and colleagues (2014) outline many of the specific mineral concentrations that appear adequate in supporting ferrets and preventing deficiencies. Calcium and phosphorus and their ratio have been studied in growing ferrets where calcium concentrations ranged from 0.6% to 0.8% of DM with calcium to phosphorus ratios of either 1.3:1 or 1:1.3.[28] Authors did not find differences in growth and concluded that, at least for short periods of time, an inverse calcium to phosphorus ratio did not yield adverse effects. Generally, a calcium to phosphorus ratio of 1.5 to 2:1 is recommended for ferrets.[5]

A recent study specifically evaluated trace mineral concentrations of commercial ferret diets and found ratios of zinc and copper may be less than ideal compared to the National Research Council (NRC) requirements. Findings that ferret diets on the market contained more than 6 times the copper recommendation for cats and mink and more than 3 times the zinc recommendation postulated a connection between diet and copper-associated hepatopathy.[29] The ratio of zinc and copper, arguably a factor just as important as pure concentrations, was also highlighted as analyzed ratios were half (6.7) the ratio suggested by the NRCs (11–13:1).[15,25,29] Minimally, these authors highlight a need for research pertaining to maximum cutoff levels of key nutrients as well as digestibility data for different trace mineral sources in ferret diets. Some folks, particularly pet parents, voice concerns about salt being added to commercial diets only as a palant to drive food consumption. However, most commercial diets contain 0.5% to 1% salt to meet the sodium and chloride requirements.

Commercial ferret diets

For decades, ferrets were fed commercial cat diets. However, in recent years, realizations that cat foods tend to be lower in protein and contain too many plant-based ingredients have led to the development of more ferret-specific diets. There is discussion around what format of food is best for ferrets, much of which centers around dental health. Both kibble and canned food can have negative implications on dental health, while raw/fresh/whole prey diets come with a high price tag and considerations for human health. Thus, a combination of dietary formats is often considered ideal to meet all physical and psychological requirements.[7,9]

Fresh, raw, freeze-dried, or whole prey diets are the most biologically appropriate for ferrets. From a manufacturing and nutritional perspective, they do not have to contain the starchy ingredients extruded foods need and can rely almost exclusively on animal-based ingredients. They can also result in lower fecal volume and odor due to high digestibility.[6,7,9] However, the price tag or potential for microbiological contamination (more so for humans preparing the diet) deters many from considering this a feasible option on its own.[7,9] Canned foods technically also need less starch and binding properties for manufacture. However, potential dental health implications of plaque accumulation[6] and dental calculi[30] along with low caloric density due to high moisture content do not bode well as a sole option for ferret diets. Extruded or pelleted foods tend to be the most popular option among current ferret owners. Longer shelf-life and ease of logistics make dry foods appealing but the hardness of kibbles can promote excessive dental wear, tartar, gingivitis, and, potentially, disease.[31] As stated earlier, a combination of diets and formats is commonly suggested for health and palatability.

Offering a variety of diets and formats from an early age can help ease of changing or altering the diet later in life.[16] Ferrets have historically been thought difficult to transition to new diets, but understanding of ferret preference and behavior can be helpful. The early and strong development of the olfactory system means ferrets can develop preferences early in life, hence the importance of introducing a variety of tastes, textures, and smells when animals are young. Also helpful to know when considering transitioning a pet ferret is the aversion, or minimally lack of preference, to fish-based diets. Ferrets do not prefer the fish flavor or aroma and tend to opt for chicken-based diets.[6,7] Liver ingredients also tend to be quite palatable to ferrets but should be limited due to high vitamin A concentrations. Fish-based diets typically contain higher PUFA concentrations making them more susceptible to oxidation. Feeding large proportions of whole, frozen, and thawed fish may lead to a thiamine deficiency due to high thiaminase activity in fish and diet of only salted fish leads to salt poisoning in ferrets.[5]

When shopping for or researching ferret foods, there is a lot to consider. Things such as format, cost, and availability should all be considered. Once you are in the pet store isle or website, here are some things to look for on the container of food.

Diet do's

- High protein – 35% to 40% DMB
  - It is particularly important to convert to a DMB when looking at canned food
  - To calculate DMB, divide the protein percentage on the bag/can by the dry matter content (100-moisture %)
  - Example: Protein: 10%, Moisture: 75%
    - Dry matter: 100 to 75 = 25%
    - Protein on a DMB: 10/0.25 = 40%
- High fat – 15% to 20% DMB
  - Also consider protein-to-fat ratio (protein/fat) and target approximately 2:1
- Low starch – less than 5% DMB
  - This will not be listed on the GA so look for the absence of high starch ingredients such as corn, potatoes, and peas.
- First 3 to 5 ingredients animal-derived
  - The source and quality of protein and fat must also be considered but are not as easy to assess on a pet food package. Look for little to no plant-based protein and fat as it is not as easily digested and utilized by ferrets. Low-quality meat meals (by-product meals) also contain indigestible protein and lack sufficient amounts of essential amino acids and should be avoided in high quantities. Ingredients are listed on pet food packaging in the order of descending inclusion, which can be used to generally assess ingredient amounts.

Diet don'ts

- A lot of plant-based ingredients, especially plant proteins
  - Plant-based ingredients are less digestible for ferrets and plant-based proteins lack sufficient levels of many amino acids ferrets need. Beware that plant-based proteins can increase the protein level on the GA but are not as beneficial as animal proteins.

- Starchy ingredients
  - Ingredients such as potatoes, corn, and peas are quite high in starch, which ferrets are not designed to digest.
- Fruit or sugary ingredients
  - While these sweet tasting ingredients are very palatable to ferrets, they are inappropriate in the diet of an obligate carnivore as they can cause digestive upset and swings in blood sugar.

Analysis of currently available ferret foods that support health, growth, and reproduction are listed in **Table 2**.

Treats and supplements

For healthy ferrets on a high-quality diet, treats and supplements are not nutritionally necessary. They can, however, provide variety and nutritional enrichment but no more than 10% of daily calories should come from treats and supplements.[6] Differing formats of treats can also be beneficial to target dental health and expose ferrets to different taste, textures, and smells. The same guidelines for choosing commercial diets apply to treats and supplements. They should be high in protein and fat, low in fiber, contain mostly animal-derived ingredients, and avoid plant-based ingredients including starchy vegetables and any fruits. Ferrets do have an intact sweet receptor gene (Tas1r2), meaning they can taste sweet, and they prefer fructose over other sugars.[32] Because ferrets prefer the naturally occurring sugar of fruits, they are highly palatable, however, as mentioned previously the high sugar content of fruits should be avoided.

Simple, meat-based commercial ferret treats can be beneficial for offering variety and building the human-animal bond. Many homemade treats can be used as well. These include chicken, cooked eggs, organ meats (avoid large quantities of liver due to high vitamin A concentrations), meat baby foods, and whole prey items. High-fat or high-calorie supplements such as Ferretone (8-in-1, Spectrum Brands, Inc, Islandia, NY, www.eightinonepet.com) and Nutri-Cal (Tomlyn Veterinary Science, Fort Worth, TX, www.tomlyn.com) can also be used in very small amounts as supplements or to aid in food transitions or administering medications.[6]

Life stages

Ferrets are generally considered young and growing kits until 1 year of age. Young ferrets have an even shorter transit time than adults, with food remaining in the digestive tract for as little as 1 hour.[6,7,16] This coupled with the rapid growth, more than quadrupling their weight between 4 and 9 weeks of age,[6] further necessitates a highly digestible diet that is calorically dense. Kits should be fed diets that contain no less than 35% protein and 20% fat DMB, which should be available at all times.[7] If acceptance of solid food is low in young or newly weaned ferrets, dry kibble can be softened with warm water, cooked eggs, and small amount of fish oil.[7] Breeding and gestating ferrets also require very high-quality diets with ample protein and calories. Protein should not be less than 35% DMB for breeding jills and in the last trimester of pregnancy her food intake will increase.[16] Lactating jills require the most calories, which can double or triple from maintenance. A high-quality food and fresh water should be provided at all times and the same softened kibble with added protein and fat described above for kits can be offered to lactating jills.[7] Currently, most commercially available foods are marketed for young, growing, and breeding ferrets and high-quality foods (listed in **Table 2**) can support all life stages with some additional supplementation.

Ferrets are considered senior or geriatric at 3 to 4 years of age. As with many carnivores, a lower protein diet (<35% DMB) can be considered for senior animals to avoid

Table 2
Analysis of commercial diets (dry matter basis) that support growth and reproduction in ferrets

	Diet A	Diet B	Diet C	Diet D	Diet E
Crude Protein %	41.5	43.3	43.2	39.5	53.0
Crude Fat %	21.1	22.8	22.7	25.2	22.6
Protein: fat Ratio	2.0	1.9	1.9	1.6	2.4
Crude Fiber %	2.3	2.9	4.5	1.5	1.6
Moisture %	4.2	10.0	12.0	7.5	7.4
Ash %	7.7	7.2	8.5	7.0	11.5
Carbohydrate %	27.3	23.8	19.9	26.8	11.3
Taurine %	0.3	0.3	0.6	0.3	0.8
Linoleic acid %	3.1	3.1	3.4	4.9	4.3
Calcium %	1.3	1.6	1.6	1.4	2.3
Phosphorus %	1.1	1.4	1.5	1.0	1.4
Ca/P ratio	1.1	1.1	1.1	1.5	1.6
Potassium %	0.8	0.6	0.8	0.7	1.1
Magnesium %	0.1	0.1	0.1	0.1	0.1
Sodium %	0.6	0.4	0.5	0.5	0.7
Iron ppm (mg/kg)	375.8	355.6	346.6	259.5	348.1
Copper mg/kg	31.3	26.7	25.0	25.9	32.9
Manganese mg/kg	73.1	80.0	85.2	86.5	77.4
Zinc mg/kg	151.4	257.8	267.0	259.5	225.0
Zn:Cu	4.8	9.7	10.7	10.0	6.8
Iodine mg/kg	2.7	2.2	2.2	2.2	2.9
Selenium mg/kg	0.3	0.7	0.2	0.4	0.9
A (IU/kg)	36,639	27,889	36,097	27,027	20,723
D3 (IU/kg)	2296	4111	4045	1946	2925
E (IU/kg)	162	278	267	324	416
K (ppm, mg/kg)	1.3	3.6	3.4	2.2	0.3
Thiamine mg/kg	13.4	62.2	61.4	48.6	58.0
Riboflavin mg/kg	26.1	22.2	25.0	59.5	13.9
Niacin mg/kg	99.2	122.2	145.5	129.7	102.4
Pantothenic acid mg/kg	26.1	29.1	28.4	37.8	51.2
Folic acid mg/kg	1.6	4.8	5.0	3.2	7.3
Pyridoxine mg/kg	13.0	19.4	31.8	37.8	12.3
Biotin mg/kg	0.6	0.5	0.5	11.0	1.3
Metabolizable Energy kcal/g	4.1	4.4	4.8	4.7	4.2

Diet A: Marshall Premium Ferret (Marshall Pet Products, North Rose, NY, www.marshallpet.com).
Diet B: Purina High Density Ferret Lab Diet 5L14 (Lab Diet, St Louis, MO, www.labdiet.com).
Diet C: Mazuri Ferret (PMI Nutrition International LLC, brentwood, MO, www.mazuri.com/.product_pdfs/5M08.pdf).
Diet D: Totally Ferret Active Show & Pet Formula (Performance Foods, Inc, Broomfield, CO, www.performancefoodsinc.net).
Diet E: Oxbow Essentials Ferret Food (Oxbow Animal Health, Omaha, NE, www.oxbowanimalhealth.com).
Adapted from Johnson-Delaney CA. Ferret nutrition. Vet Clin North Am Exot Anim Pract 2014;17(3):449 to 470. https://doi.org/10.1016/j.cvex.2014.05.008; with permission.

kidney issues and strain, but depending on health and body condition, this might not be necessary. Weight loss and muscle wasting can occur in senior ferrets, potentially due to a declining olfactory system and reduced food consumption, so more frequent feedings are recommended so food does not become stale and lose its scent.[20] There are now commercial senior ferret foods on the market but a drastic diet change with an older animal may not be successful and benefits and dietary evaluation should be done carefully.

Clinical Illness with Nutritional Implications

Any illness or disease in ferrets can require nutritional support as resulting anorexia can contribute to hepatic lipidosis or hypoglycemia.[33] Assist feeding of meat-based canned/soft diets or meat baby food can be beneficial if the animal will accept them. For animals that will not eat canned or soft foods, high-calorie gels or pastes (Ferretone, Nutri-Cal) can be used on a short-term basis to supplement calories. For longer term assist feedings solutions, nutritionally complete options should be utilized such as Critical Care Carnivore (Oxbow Animal Health, Omaha, NE, www.oxbowanimalhealth.com) or Intensive Care Carnivore (EmerAid, Cornell, IL, www.emeraid.com). Some illnesses and diseases are more closely tied to nutrition and have more specific outcomes or goals.

Gastrointestinal

Gastroenteritis is common in ferrets and although its exact cause is largely unknown, a dietary correlation has been theorized. Dietary intolerance or sensitivity, particularly to high-starch/carbohydrate diets or certain protein sources (though neither been proven), has historically been thought to be associated with inflammatory bowel disease (IBD) in ferrets.[31] A high-protein, low-carbohydrate diet is always recommended, and novel or hydrolyzed protein diets may be necessary with ferrets diagnosed with IBD. Because nearly all available ferret diets are chicken-based, novel protein cat foods can be used, though Totally Ferret does offer a turkey, venison, and lamb ferret diet (Performance Foods, Broomfield, CO, www.totallyferret.com) that can be used as a novel protein food.[31] Animals, including ferrets, with chronic diarrhea have been shown to have low cobalamin levels, so vitamin B12 supplementation may be beneficial in ferrets with IBD if serum concentrations suggest.[20] Hoppes (2010) recommended cobalamin therapy extrapolated from cats with 250 µg subcutaneously weekly for 6 weeks, followed by 250 µg every other week for 6 weeks, then once monthly.

Insulinoma

One of the most common ailments diagnosed in pet ferrets is insulinoma.[7] These insulin-secreting beta cell tumors can lead to hypoglycemia by rendering a ferret unable to regulate insulin production. To combat low blood glucose and address this disease, surgery to remove tumors is often, and most successfully, coupled with dietary intervention.[34] Dietary considerations in ferrets with insulinoma include ad libitum access to a very high-quality food (high protein and fat, low carbohydrate) to regulate and control blood glucose dip and spikes. Treats high in fat and protein are also often recommended especially in association with activity of animals or in between meals.

Urolithiasis

Urolithiasis in ferrets has been an issue receiving growing interest and investigation over the past several years. Struvite urolithiasis was once the most common form and thought to originate from high plant protein diets.[1,35–37] However, from 1992 to 2009, the number of cystine urolith submissions at the Minnesota Urolith Center increased more than 10-fold[38] and cystine uroliths are now considered the most common among domestic ferrets in North America.[35] Interestingly, this trend does not seem to hold true in the European ferret population.[39]

In normal metabolism, cystine is filtered in the glomerulus of the kidneys then reabsorbed from the proximal renal tubules from the urine. In dogs and humans, a genetic defect of the renal tubules affects reabsorption and contributes to the development of cystinuria.[35] A genetic component in ferrets is thought to contribute to cystine urolithiasis, though this has not been proven and etiology of cysteine urolithiasis in ferrets is still largely unknown. The mean age of onset for ferrets with cysteine uroliths is 3 to 4 years, which some authors argue would be earlier if caused by a genetic disorder.[38] Furthermore, neutered male ferrets seem to be more predisposed, likely due to the size and anatomy of the urethra.[38,39]

Cystine is composed of two cysteine amino acids joined by a disulfide bond. In addition to dietary sources of cysteine and cystine directly, cysteine can be made from methionine within the body. Cystine is relatively insoluble, especially in acidic urine.[35] General recommendations for dietary treatment of cystine urolithiasis in humans are to reduce urinary cystine excretion and increase cystine solubility by increasing fluid intake, restricting dietary protein, and restrict dietary sodium.[40]

For ferrets, a diet high in cereals and plant-based ingredients in theory should be beneficial as they alkalinize the urine, thereby increasing the solubility of cystine,[35] but this is not the case. It is generally noted that animal proteins contain more cysteine than cereal and legumes.[41,42] However, data from analysis of peas show concentrations of 1.25% to 1.52% cysteine (DMB) while chicken ingredients used in pet foods ranged from 0.36% to 0.69% cysteine (DMB).[43–45] Other authors suggest that plant proteins such as legumes may lead to higher levels of cystine in the urine, though this seems to be mostly theoretic.[35] Anecdotally, many veterinary clinics report a correlation between increased incidence of cystine uroliths and diets containing peas or lentils.[35] One recent case-controlled study did find that ferrets with cystine urolithiasis were nearly 58 times more likely to receive a grain-free diet compared to the reference population, though causation could not be drawn from the study.[39] Interestingly, Lamglait and colleagues (2021) found that grain-free diets, 83% of which contained peas and legumes, were not higher in cysteine concentrations compared to non–grain-free diets. Of ferrets with uroliths that were originally fed a grain-free diet, after surgical removal, 6 ferrets that transitioned to non–grain-free diets did not experience reoccurrence while 2 ferrets that remained on a grain-free diet had uroliths less than a year later. It is important to note, however, that not all ferrets on a grain-free diet had uroliths and 2 of the 36 urolith cases were fed a non–grain-free diet, further indicating a multifactorial etiology.

The high protein requirement of ferrets does not aid in the treatment of cystine urolithiasis as high-protein diets only acidify urine.[36] Until further research is conducted in ferrets, practical treatments to avoid cystine urolithiasis include encouraging water intake, controlling sodium levels, monitoring methionine and cystine in the diet, and increasing urine alkalinity via potassium citrate.[35,37] The inclusion of high-quality canned diets can also be used to encourage water intake as they typically contain between 70% and 80% moisture. The use of alkalinating agents should always be discussed and closely monitored.

FUTURE RESEARCH

More research regarding legume-containing diets and the genetic component of cystine urolithiasis is clearly indicated. Controlled, long-term studies with dietary treatments are needed to fully evaluate the impact of certain diets and dietary ingredients.

Further research to elucidate the exact nutrient requirements of ferrets should also be a focus. This research should highlight not just dietary minimum and maximum inclusions, but optimal concentrations and ratios of dietary nutrients for long-term ferret health.

SUMMARY

Pet ferrets have been domesticated for thousands of years, but ideal feeding practices in captivity are still being determined. Their short and simple digestive tract along with exclusively prey diet in the wild highlights the need for a high-protein and fat, low-carbohydrate diet. The difficulty of manufacturing a diet like this has been an issue. Extruded, canned, and raw/freeze-dried are popular options on the market today, but balancing price point, nutritional adequacy, and dental health is not straightforward. It is recommended that ferret diets consist of all these formats to introduce variety, nutritional adequacy, and healthy balance. The exact nutritional requirements of these animals deserve more attention to elucidate the exact needs including ideal protein and fat concentrations, mineral maximums and ratios, as well as vitamin inclusions for long-term health. Impacts of life stage, particularly senior animals, should also be evaluated. Studies evaluating nutritional and diet impacts on certain common health issues and disease are warranted. Nutritional implications theorized to impact health status, such as carbohydrates in IBD and grain-free or legumes in cystine urolithiasis, should be thoroughly investigated to determine best feeding practices.

CLINICS CARE POINTS

- High protein (35%–40% DMB) and fat (20% DMB) diets should always be recommended and fed to ferrets.
- Protein-to-fat ratios should be evaluated in commercially available ferret diets as more protein is not always better and should be balanced with fat at an approximate ratio of 2:1.
- Low carbohydrate (<20%) and starch (<5%) diets are best digested and support ferret gastrointestinal health.
- Plant ingredients, particularly plant-based proteins, are not well utilized by ferrets and may lack the amino acid profile they require.
- Plant-derived ingredients should be minimal in any ferret food.
- Fruits in foods or used as snacks can be detrimental as ferrets love the taste of fructose and may prefer that to any other food if given too often.

DISCLOSURE

Author was previously employed with Oxbow Animal Health and developed the Essentials Ferret Food.

REFERENCES

1. Wolf TM. Ferrets. In: Mitchell MA, Tully TN, editors. Manual of exotic pet practice. St. Louis: W.B. Saunders; 2009. p. 345–74. https://doi.org/10.1016/B978-141600 119-5.50016-0.
2. Boyce SW, Zingg BM, Lightfoot TL. Behavior of *Mustela putorius furo* (the domestic ferret). Vet Clin North Am Exot Anim Pract 2001;4(3):697–712.

3. Ball RS. Issues to consider for preparing ferrets as research subjects in the laboratory. ILAR J 2006;47(4):348–57.
4. Evans H, Quoc An N. Anatomy of the ferret. In: Fox JG, Marini RP, editors. Biology and diseases of the ferret. Ames: John Wiley & Sons Inc.; 2014. p. 23–67. https://doi.org/10.1002/9781118782699.ch2.
5. Fox JG, Schultz CS, Boler BMV. Nutrition of the ferret. In: Fox JG, Marini RP, editors. Biology and diseases of the ferret. Ames: John Wiley & Sons Inc.; 2014. p. 123–43. https://doi.org/10.1002/9781118782699.ch5.
6. Bell JA. Ferret nutrition. Vet Clin North Am Exot Anim Pract 1999;2(1):169–92.
7. Johnson-Delaney CA. Ferret nutrition. Vet Clin North Am Exot Anim Pract 2014; 17(3):449–70.
8. Dessem D, Druzinsky RE. Jaw-muscle activity in ferrets, *Mustela putorius furo.* J Morphol 1992;213(2):275–86.
9. Bullen LE. Nutrtion for pocket pets (ferrets, rabbits, and rodents). Vet Clin Small Anim 2021;51:583–604.
10. Sundling L, Ahlstrøm O, Tauson AH. Comparative digestibility of nutrients and energy in ferrets (*Mustela putorius furo*), mink (*Neovison vison*) and cats (*Felis catus*). In: Larsen PF, Møller SH, Clausen T, editors. Proceedings of the xth international scientific congress in Fur animal production, vol. 36. Wageningen, Netherlands: Wageningen Academic Publishers; 2012. p. 112–20.
11. Smith GP, Ragg JR, Waldrup KA, et al. Diet of feral ferrets (*Mustela furo*) from pastoral habitats in otago and southland, New Zealand. New Zeal J Zool 1995;22(4): 363–9.
12. Ragg JR. Intraspecific and seasonal differences in the diet of feral ferrets (*Mustela furo*) in a pastoral habitat, East Otago, New Zealand. N Z J Ecol 1998;22(2): 113–9.
13. Dierenfeld ES, Alcorn HL, Jacobsen KL. Nutrient composition of whole vertebrate prey (exclusing fish) fed in zoos. National Agricultural Library; 2002. http://www.nal.usda.gov/awic/zoo/WholePreyFinal02May29.pdf.
14. Matchett CA, Marr R, Berard FM, et al. The laboratory ferret. In: Suckow MA, editor. The laboratory animal pocket reference series. Boca Raton: CRC Press; 2012.
15. National Research Council (NRC). Nutrient requirements of mink and foxes. Second Rev. Washington, DC: National Academies Press; 1982. https://doi.org/10.17226/1114.
16. Kupersmith DS. A practical overview of small mammal nutrition. Semin Avian Exot Pet Med 1998;7(3):141–7.
17. Zhang HH, Li GY, Ren EJ, et al. Effects of diets with different protein and dl-methionine levels on the growth performance and N-balance of growing minks. J Anim Physiol Anim Nutr 2012;96(3):436–41.
18. Devendra R, Deshmukh TCS. Arginine requirement and ammonia toxicity in ferrets. J Nutr 1983;113(8):1664–7.
19. Emudianughe TS, Caldwell J, Smith RL. The utilization of exogenous taurine for the conjugation of xenobiotic acids in the ferret. Xenobiotica 1983;13(3):133–8.
20. Hoppes SM. The senior rerret (*Mustela putorius furo*). Vet Clin North Am Exot Anim Pract 2010;13(1):107–22.
21. Atwater WO, Bryant AP. The availability and fuel value of food materials. Rep. Storrs Agr. Exp. Sta 1900;73.
22. Dinicolantonio JJ, O'Keefe JH. Importance of maintaining a low omega-6/omega-3 ratio for reducing inflammation. Open Hear 2018;5(2):3–6.
23. Association of American Feed Control Officials. Official Publication. Atlanta: AAFCO, Inc., 2023.

24. Raila J, Gomez C, Schweigert FJ. The ferret as a model for vitamin A metabolism in carnivores. J Nutr 2002;132(6 SUPPL. 1):1787–9.
25. National Research Council (NRC). Nutrient requirements of dogs and cats. 1st edition. Washington, DC: National Academies Press; 2006.
26. Brooks HV, Rammell CG, Hoogenboom JJL, et al. Observations on an outbreak of nutritional steatitis (yellow fat disease) in fitch (*Mustella putorius furo*). N Z Vet J 1985;33(9):141–5.
27. Manning DD, Bell JA. Derivation of gnotobiotic ferrets: perinatal diet and hand-rearing requirements. Lab Anim Sci 1990;40(1):51–5.
28. Edfors C, Ullrey DE, Aulerich RJ. Effects of dietary calcium concentration and calcium-phosphorus ratio on growth and selected plasma and bone measures in young European ferrets (*Mustela putorius furo*). J Zoo Wildl Med 1990;21(2): 185–91.
29. Torkelson MR, Heinze CR, Graham JE. Survey of copper and zinc concentrations in commercially available dry ferret diets. J Exot Pet Med 2022;42:6–10.
30. Harper DS, Mann PH, Regnier S. Measurement of dietary and dentifrice effects upon calculus accumulation rates in the domestic ferret. J Dent Res 1990;69(2): 447–50.
31. Hoefer HL, Fox JG, Bell JA. Gastrointestinal diseases of ferrets. In: Quesenberry KE, Orcutt CJ, Mans C, et al, editors. Ferrets, rabbits, and rodents: clinical medicine and surgery. 4th edition. St. Louis, MO: Elsevier; 2020. p. 27–45. https://doi.org/10.1016/B978-1-4160-6621-7.00003-8.
32. Li X, Glaser D, Li W, et al. Analyses of sweet receptor gene (Tas1r2) and prefer-ence for sweet stimuli in species of carnivora. J Hered 2009;100(Supplement 1): S90–100.
33. de Matos REC, Morrisey JK. Common procedures in the pet ferret. Vet Clin North Am Exot Anim Pract 2006;9(2):347–65.
34. Rosenthal KL, Wyre NR. Endocrine diseases of ferrets. In: Quesenberry KE, Orcutt CJ, Mans C, et al, editors. Ferrets, rabbits, and rodents: clinical medicine and surgery. 4th edition. St. Louis, MO: Elsevier; 2020. p. 86–102. https://doi.org/10.1016/B978-1-4160-6621-7.00007-5.
35. Pacheco RE. Cystine urolithiasis in ferrets. Vet Clin North Am Exot Anim Pract 2020;23(2):309–19.
36. Orcutt CJ. Ferret urogenital diseases. Vet Clin North Am Exot Anim Pract 2003; 6(1):113–38.
37. Fisher PG. Exotic companion mammal urolithiasis. 2015. Available at: https://newcms.eventkaddy.net/event_data/60/session_files/AV026_Conference_Note_jjacobs_cvma.net_AV026_FISHER_ExoticCompanionMammalUrolithiasis_2015 0511175206.pdf. Accessed March 14, 2023.
38. Nwaokorie EE, Osborne CA, Lulich JP, et al. Epidemiological evaluation of cystine urolithiasis in domestic ferrets (*Mustela putorius furo*): 70 cases (1992–2009). J Am Vet Med Assoc 2013;242(8):1099–103.
39. Lamglait B, Brieger A, Rainville MP, et al. Retrospective case control study of pet ferrets with cystine urolithiasis in Quebec, Canada: Epidemiological and clinical features. J Vet Med Surg 2021;5(1):31.
40. Siener R, Bitterlich N, Birwé H, et al. The impact of diet on urinary risk factors for cystine stone formation. Nutrients 2021;13(2):1–10.
41. Ismail NI, Hashim YZH, Jamal P, et al. Production of cysteine: Approaches, chal-lenges and potential solution. Int J Biotechnol Wellness Ind 2014;3(3):95–101.
42. Larsson SC, Håkansson N, Wolk A. Dietary cysteine and other amino acids and stroke incidence in women. Stroke 2015;46(4):922–6.

43. Witten S, Böhm H, Aulrich K. Effect of variety and environment on the contents of crude nutrients, lysine, methionine and cysteine in organically produced field peas (*Pisum sativum L.*) and field beans (*Vicia faba L.*). Appl Agric Forestry Res 2015;65(3–4):205–16.
44. Evans IM, Boulter D. Crude protein and sulphur amino acid contents of some commercial varieties of peas and beans. J Sci Food Agric 1980;31(3):238–42.
45. Oba PM, Utterback PL, Parsons CM, et al. Chemical composition, true nutrient digestibility, and true metabolizable energy of chicken-based ingredients differing by processing method using the precision-fed cecectomized rooster assay. J Anim Sci 2019;97(3):998–1009.

Insectivore Nutrition – A Review of Current Knowledge

Breanna P. Modica, MS, MPhil*, Elizabeth A. Koutsos, PhD

KEYWORDS

- Insect • Insectivore • Diet • Nutrition • Captive management

KEY POINTS

- Insectivorous animals are represented in virtually all taxa, and insects may be a primary or partial component of the diet.
- Determination of optimal nutrient requirements for insectivores requires the integration of data from various domesticated species.
- The number of insects available in free-ranging animal diets cannot be replicated for animals under captive management.
- A combination of insects (with appropriate supplementation), formulated feeds, and supplementary food items is often the best option for nutritional and behavioral management of insectivores in human care.

INTRODUCTION

Insects are "the most abundant and diverse animal group on Earth"[1] making it no surprise that varying degrees of insectivory, or insect consumption, are present across numerous species of mammals, birds, reptiles, amphibians, and fish. Insectivores play an important role in the balance of insect biomass across ecosystems. There are over 400 identified species of mammals (in the order Insectivora, although this order is currently disputed) and birds reported to purposefully ingest insects in the wild. In addition, at least 100 reptile species and most amphibians have been identified as facultative or obligate insectivores.[2–5] Estimates regarding the total number of insectivorous fish species are currently unknown. This review is focused on terrestrial vertebrate insectivore species for which more information is currently known. The goal of this review is to summarize current knowledge of insectivore nutrition, not to provide specific feeding and nutrient requirements for a given species. The authors suggest reviewing species-specific information whenever possible.

Insectivores are classified by preferred consumption of invertebrate prey, which are defined by a lack of bony skeleton. Invertebrates include insects, arachnids, worms,

EnviroFlight, LLC, 2100 Production Drive, Apex, NC 27539, USA
* Corresponding author. 2100 Production Drive Apex, NC 27539.
E-mail address: bpmodica@outlook.com

Vet Clin Exot Anim 27 (2024) 47–69
https://doi.org/10.1016/j.cvex.2023.07.003

crustaceans, and mollusks. There are two main classifications of insectivores derived from the proportion of the diet that is invertebrate-based; obligate insectivores subsist on an entirely invertebrate diet, at least in their free-ranging habitats. This class includes animals such as anteater and tamandua species, *Myrmecophaga tridactyla* and *Tamandua tetradactyla*.[6,7] Facultative insectivores, in their free-ranging habitat, subsist on invertebrate-based diets augmented with other food items. Regardless of the degree of insectivory in their free-ranging habitats, in captively managed situations, these species must be fed different diet components and in different proportions. This is due to the fact that wild-type insect species are generally not available as a food source in zoos and aquaria, because we are lacking complete information on free-ranging diets for many species, and because captively managed animals likely have some differing nutrient requirements due to environmental conditions, energy expenditure and other life history traits.

INSECTIVORE NUTRITION
Digestive Anatomy

When considering the feeding of captively managed insectivores, it is important to consider their method of procuring diet items. Insectivores have adapted very diverse, but efficient ways to catch and digest their target prey items. For example, birds can catch insects during flight, reptiles often stalk and hunt insects, and some mammals are able to use specialized methods such as echolocation to find and capture insect prey. Adaptation of mouthparts for specialized capture and ingestion of insects marks the start of the insectivore digestive tract. The tongue may be long (as seen in anteaters, chameleons, some horned lizards, etc.) and anchored farther back in the mouth, or even to the sternum.[8,9] This allows for rapid prehension of precise invertebrate prey types. The tongue of some insectivores is coated with mucus or saliva that protects the animal from potentially toxic prey.[10] For example, the short-tailed shrew (*Blarina brevicauda*) produces saliva that is toxic to its insect prey.[10] Salivary glands may also be enlarged.[11] Dentition is also adapted with some insectivores lacking any (such as anteaters, echidnas, and pangolins), some insectivores having reduced dentition (such as armadillos), some having unusual dentition (such as columnar cheek teeth in aardvarks), some having large dentition (such as bats consuming beetles), and some having small dentition (such as bats consuming moths).[8,11,12]

After the mouth, most insectivore digestive tracts continue to a thick-walled simple stomach containing some type of grinding function to accommodate mechanical reduction of particle size. Rocks have been reported in feces of wild anteaters and are thought to be intentionally ingested to support this grinding function.[8] The small and large intestines are also simple and largely unseparated with some insectivores having a cecum, although its functionality is not well known. It has been demonstrated from fecal samples of captively managed primates that gut microbiota includes significantly higher counts of Bifidobacteria in facultative insectivorous species (frugivore-insectivores, 19% and gummivore-insectivores, 12%) as compared to that of non-insectivorous primates (frugivore-folivores, 4% and frugivore-omnivores, 2%).[13] While bifidobacteria are known to be involved in carbohydrate metabolism and utilize many dietary carbohydrate sources that escape digestion in the small intestine, two Bifidobacteria (*B. pseudocatenulatum* and *B. longum*) have expressed high binding affinity specific to chitin.[13,14] Furthermore, *Bifidobacterium animalis* were reported to multiply by almost six times in the human gut when cricket (*Gryllodes sigillatus*) powder was part of the diet.[15] This change was attributed to the main dietary difference of chitin present in the cricket treatment.[15] These data indicate the chitin-digesting potential of Bifidobacteria. Information on overall digestive efficiencies in insectivores is limited but mean retention time, crude protein and lipid digestibility in captive ant-eaters has been reported as similar to domestic dogs and cats, which is not unexpected based on physical digestive tract similarities.[8]

Other adaptations possessed by insectivores may include an acute sense of hearing or smell. The aye-aye (*Daubentonia madagascariensis*) will tap logs and use the percussive feedback to locate insects, while the short-beaked echidna (*Tachyglossus aculeatus*) uses acute smell achieved by an extensively folded olfactory bulb and nasal passages covered in olfactory epithelium to enhance olfaction.[7,16] Some insectivores have large well-defined claws or long digits that help claw into insect nests or reach into small insect tunnels.[8,11] For example, the third finger of the aye-aye is its longest digit while the fourth finger of the striped possum (*Dactylopsila trivirgata*) is the longest. Unique to a few species are the prey-locating abilities of echolocation (some bats) and electroreception (echidna). Insectivorous bat species are capable of both oral and nasal echolocation, with nasal echolocation allowing them to ingest prey and continue to echolocate simultaneously.[17] Echidnas (*Tachyglossus*, *Ornithorhynchus*, and *Zaglossus*) are one of the only three mammals with electroreception abilities, the other two being the platypus (*Ornithorhynchus anatinus*) and the Guiana dolphin (*Sotalia guianensis*).[18] Electroreception is the detection of electrical signals produced by living animals and is restricted to aquatic environments where water possesses the low electrical resistivity required for the movement and detection of electrical currents.[18] Electroreception is much more developed in *Zaglossus* echidnas that are native to humid environments where moisture in the soil provides the necessary conductivity.[19] Lastly, there are tactile adaptations such as Eimer's organ, on the nose of moles (Talpidae).[20,21] This organ is highly innervated and helps moles find invertebrate prey underground.[21]

It is known that free-ranging insectivores generally have a much more varied diet than is possible for their captively managed counterparts. For example, observations of the diets of free-ranging meerkats (*Suricata suricatta*) revealed an average of 6.7 ± 1.1 different prey categories ingested daily with insects accounting for 78.1% of prey, the diet of free-ranging Chinese pangolins (*Manis pentadactyla*) includes eight species of ants and eight species of termites, while it has been reported that many wild insectivorous bird species frequently consume combinations of seven main arthropod orders including araneae, coleoptera, diptera, hemiptera, hymenoptera, lepidoptera, and orthoptera.[4,22,23] In comparison, captive insectivores are often provided no more than three different types of insect prey (most commonly crickets and mealworms) due to limited availability of feeder insects.[24,25] Furthermore, some insectivores must hunt frequently and ingest a large number of insects in order to fulfill their nutritional and energetic requirements.[26] For example, a single little brown bat (*Myotis lucifugus*) can ingest up to 1200 mosquitos in 1 hour.[1] Frequent feedings are also required for insectivores consuming insect species that include defensive individuals ("soldiers") that attack predators relatively quickly upon a disturbance, such as ants and termites.[8] Insectivores are also able to adjust to seasonal variability of available insect species as well as adjust consumption amounts during certain life stages, such as breeding seasons.[1,27,28] Organic matter may also be ingested with invertebrates and may provide a critical source of mineral nutrition. For example, captive anteaters have been reported to consume an average of 93.0 g of soil per day.[8]

Natural feeding habits and nutritional requirements of insectivore species are not completely known; therefore, recommendations are often highly generalized based on research in model species. For example, it has been reported that anteater digestive anatomy and physiology resemble that of domestic dogs and cats indicating that a combination of omnivorous and carnivorous nutrient requirements may be appropriate proxies for these insectivorous mammals.[8] However, energy requirements may vary from domesticated model species. Basal metabolic rates of insectivorous mammals (>100 g BW) and reptiles tend to be lower than carnivorous species, while BMR of insectivorous birds tend to be similar to carnivorous species. Estimated energy requirements and feed intake of free-ranging animal species with varying insectivorous tendencies commonly kept in zoologic institutions or as pets are provided in **Table 1**. It is recommended to provide approximately 75% of free-ranging energy requirements to animals in captivity as they typically experience lower energy demands than their free-ranging counterparts.

Protein

Animals require amino acids and nitrogen to synthesize non-essential amino acids. Dietary crude protein is often used a proxy for these nitrogen needs, but it is critical to evaluate the quality (ie, the amino acid composition and anticipated availability of those amino acids) when considering a target dietary crude protein content. Recommendations for dietary crude protein for domestic dogs and cats, mink, and foxes are generally in the range of 17.5% to 30.0% and may be appropriate for insectivorous mammals.[45] Higher dietary crude protein content may also be appropriate, particularly for obligate insectivores for which free-ranging dietary protein levels are generally high (on a dry matter basis, DMB). For examples, 13 insectivorous free-ranging bird species in Australia including robins, flycatchers and others consumed insects that were consistently high in protein (DMB) such as Araneae, 76.3%; Coleoptera, 73.8%; Lepidoptera, 64.4%; and Orthoptera, 68.8%.[28] These values are similar to those reported for ant species (DMB), such as *Polyrhachis vicina* Roger (64.5%, male and 64.1%, female), and *Polyrhachis lamellidens* Smith (58.6%) commonly ingested by free-ranging pangolins.[23]

Crude protein content of insects may include nitrogen in body tissue but may also include nitrogen present in the exoskeleton as chitin.[8,23] Chitin is also represented in the acid detergent fiber (ADF) fraction, complicating true chitin analysis.[46] For many insectivores, it is unknown if they synthesize the enzyme chitinase, which would allow for autoenzymatic digestion of chitin as a nitrogen and energy source, or if they possess appropriate symbiotic gut bacteria that may help digest this non-protein nitrogen source.[8,47] Acidic chitinases have been identified in chicken, pig, mouse, rat, the insectivorous common marmoset (*Callithrix jacchus*), and the insectivorous Sunda pangolin (*Manis javanica*) digestive tracts, but not in domestic dog digestive tracts.[12,48] Furthermore, acidic chitinase extracts from the common marmoset were found to degrade mealworm (*Tenebrio molitor*) exoskeletons.[48] If not completely digested, the chitin content of insects may act similarly to structural carbohydrates (fiber) in an insectivore's digestive tract and help improve fecal consistency.[8,48] Considering the presence of chitin in several insect orders ranging from 2.6% in adult Haplotaxida worms to 18.5% in adult Isoptera termites (DMB), it may be advantageous to include a low level of an insoluble fiber source, such as cellulose, in the diet of captively managed insectivores to support gut health.[7,8,11] However, chitin powder or ingredients with known chitin content, such as shrimp meal, may be a more appropriate option since cellulose and chitin are not structurally the same beyond both being carbohydrate polymers.[49] Recently, 5.0% ground food-grade chitin in the diet of Chinese pangolins was shown to improve fecal consistency.[23]

Amino acid concentrations provided by the crude protein content are a crucial consideration to meet the nutrient requirements of insectivores. While insects may provide a complete amino acid profile, methionine and cystine are often the first

Table 1
Calculated free-ranging energy requirements and feed intake of select animal species with varying insectivorous tendencies commonly kept in captivity

Common Name	Genus and Species	BW[a], g	FMR[b], kJ/d	FMI[c], G/d	DMI[d], G/d
Mammals					
Giant anteater[29]	Myrmecophaga tridactyla	27,215.5 / 45,359.2	4002.31 / 5499.22	648.67 / 891.28	214.03 / 294.08
Southern tamandua (lesser anteater)[29]	Tamandua tetradactyla	4535.92	1313.11	212.82	70.22
White-bellied pangolin[30]	Phataginus tricuspis	1678.29 / 2404.04	707.49 / 884.71	114.67 / 143.39	37.83 / 47.31
Aardvark[31]	Orycteropus afer	45,359.2 / 81,646.6	5499.22 / 7926.49	891.28 / 1284.68	294.08 / 423.88
9-Banded armadillo[32]	Xenarthra cingulata	3628.74 / 7711.07	1142.94 / 1826.59	185.24 / 296.04	61.12 / 97.68
Slender-tailed meerkat[24]	Suricata suricatta	1028.0 / 1100.0	521.57 / 544.00	84.53 / 88.17	27.89 / 29.09
Lesser Madagascar hedgehog tenrec[29]	Echinops telfairi	113.0 / 255.0	132.09 / 219.14	21.41 / 35.52	7.06 / 11.72
Greater Madagascar hedgehog tenrec[29]	Setifer setosus	180.0 / 270.0	176.46 / 227.07	28.60 / 36.80	9.44 / 12.14
Birds					
American kestrel[30]	Falco sparverius	85.0 / 170.0	222.34 / 362.44	37.43 / 61.02	12.35 / 20.14
Lesser kestrel[33]	Falco naumanni	120.0 / 140.0	283.53 / 316.08	47.73 / 53.21	15.75 / 17.56
African dwarf kingfisher[30]	Ispidina lecontei	9.0 / 12.0	45.66 / 55.92	7.69 / 9.41	2.54 / 3.11
Giant kingfisher[30]	Megaceryle maxima	490.0	764.47	128.07	42.47
Guam kingfisher[29]	Todiramphus cinnamominus	50.0 / 70.0	152.95 / 193.89	25.75 / 32.64	8.50 / 10.77
Southern ground hornbill[30]	Bucorvus leadbeateri	3447.3 / 6168.86	3024.78 / 4558.96	509.22 / 767.50	168.04 / 253.28

(continued on next page)

Table 1
(continued)

Common Name	Genus and Species	BW[a], g	FMR[b], kJ/d	FMI[c], G/d	DMI[d], G/d
Red-billed dwarf hornbill[30]	*Tockus camurus*	84.0	220.49	37.12	12.25
		115.0	275.15	46.32	15.29
Greater roadrunner[34]	*Geococcyx californianus*	340.19	591.07	99.51	32.84
Eastern screech owl[29]	*Megascops asio*	130.0	299.99	50.50	16.67
		220.0	434.69	73.18	24.15
White-fronted bee-eater[30]	*Merops bullockoides*	28.0	101.63	17.11	5.65
		39.0	128.37	21.61	7.13
Carmine bee-eater[35]	*Merops nubicus*	41.6 ± 0.85	134.35 ± 1.94	22.62 ± 0.33	7.46 ± 0.10
		48.1 ± 1.23	148.83 ± 2.70	25.06 ± 0.46	8.27 ± 0.15
Reptiles					
Leopard gecko[30]	*Eublepharis macularius*	50.0	7.00	1.18	0.39
		80.0	10.76	1.81	0.60
Crested gecko[36]	*Correlophus ciliatus*	35.0	5.05	0.85	0.28
Common inland bearded dragon[32]	*Pogona vitticeps*	453.59	52.54	9.35	2.92
Northern blue-tongue skink[32]	*Tiliqua scincoides*	481.94	55.53	9.35	3.09
Chinese water dragon[37]	*Physignathus cocincinus*	182.6 ± 101.8	22.87 ± 11.72	3.85 ± 1.97	1.27 ± 0.66
		358.8 ± 158.0	42.41 ± 17.12	7.14 ± 2.89	2.36 ± 0.95
Veiled chameleon[38]	*Chamaeleo calyptratus*	102 ± 16.8	13.43 ± 2.02	2.26 ± 0.34	0.75 ± 0.12
Panther chameleon[38]	*Furcifer pardalis*	141.8 ± 20.1	18.15 ± 2.35	3.06 ± 0.40	1.01 ± 0.13
Jackson's chameleon[39]	*Trioceros jacksonii*	37.2 ± 7.1	5.34 ± 0.94	0.90 ± 0.16	0.30 ± 0.06
Alligator lizard[40,41]	*Abronia taeniata*	16.4	2.53	0.43	0.14
Frilled lizard[42]	*Chalamydosaurus kingii*	453.59	52.54	8.85	2.92
		907.19	99.00	16.67	5.51

It is recommended to provide approximately 75% of free-ranging energy requirements to animals in captivity as they typically experience lower energy demands than their free-ranging counterparts.

[a] BW, body weight; provided as average, average ± SD, or range (sources listed later in discussion).

[b] Mammalian insectivore FMR, field metabolic rate: kJ/d = 6.98(BW, g)[0.622]. Avian insectivore FMR: kJ/d = 9.70(BW, g)[0.705]. Reptilian insectivore FMR calculated as feed intake of 0.0109 or 0.0330(BW,g)[0.914] for dry matter and fresh matter, respectively, divided by FMI conversion factor later in discussion.[43]

[c] FMI, fresh matter intake using 6.17 kJ/g for mammals and 5.94 kJ/g for birds and reptiles.[44]

[d] DMI, dry matter intake using 18.7 kJ/g for mammals and 18.0 kJ/g for birds and reptiles.[44]

limiting amino acids in insects.[50,51] Dietary methionine + cystine recommendations (DMB) across domestic dog and cat life stages range from 0.34% to 1.04% (minimum, based on a 4000 kcal ME diet).[45] For fish, birds and species without a urea cycle, other amino acids such as arginine may become more limiting.[52] Taurine, a sulfur-containing amino acid required in the diet of domestic cats is also presumed to be a requirement for obligate mammalian insectivores. Giant anteaters have presented with clinical symptoms of cardiomyopathy and low blood taurine levels. Minimum recommended dietary taurine levels for cats range from 0.1% to 0.17% (based on extruded and canned cat foods, respectively and based on a 4000 kcal ME diet), and these recommendations may be appropriate for obligate insectivores as well.[8,53] However, it is known that dietary fiber, or compounds that act as dietary fiber, can reduce the availability of dietary taurine. Clinical monitoring of whole blood taurine is recommended if dietary taurine adequacy is of concern. Taurine is naturally found in animal-derived food items. For example, raw mammalian and avian muscle meats contain average taurine levels of 444 and 337 mg/kg, respectively.[54] Taurine is also found in algae, but not from strict vegetarian food items.[45]

Lipids

A crude fat range of 5.0% to 15.0% derived from minimum crude fat recommendations for domestic dogs and cats, mink, and foxes may be appropriate for insectivorous animals.[45] Insect orders frequently consumed by 13 insectivorous free-ranging bird species in Australia were moderate in fat with average fat contents (DMB) of Araneae, 9.6%; Coleoptera, 12.0%; Lepidoptera, 12.0%; and Orthoptera, 7.4%.[28] These values are also similar to those reported for ant species (*P vicina* Roger, 9.5%, male and 8.6%, female; and *P lamellidens* Smith, 8.5%, DMB) commonly ingested by free-ranging pangolins.[23]

Linoleic acid is considered the only essential fatty acid for most mammals, while domestic cats also require arachidonic acid.[54] Minimum essential fatty acid recommendations (DMB) are 1.0% linoleic acid for dogs, 0.5% linoleic acid for cats, and 0.02% arachidonic acid for cats.[45] In general, insects appear to be good sources of linoleic acid with commercially raised black soldier fly larvae (*Hermetia illucens*) and mealworms (*T molitor*) consisting of 2.6% to 6.0% (DMB) total omega-6 fatty acids, respectively.[55] Long-chain omega-3 fatty acids may be appropriate for insectivores which consume aquatic insects in their free-ranging habitat.[56] It is important to note that insect fatty acid profiles are strongly influenced by their diets, so analysis of free-ranging insect fatty acid profiles (when available) as well as those from sourced feeder insects is important in order to match anticipated needs with dietary inputs.

Diets of free-ranging insectivores are typically lower in overall saturated fatty acids compared to that of captively managed animals, which is most likely due to higher inclusions of vertebrate-based diet items for the latter.[24] Additionally, diets of free-ranging insectivores are likely lower in cholesterol because insects are not a source of dietary cholesterol since they lack the ability to synthesize this lipid.[24,57] The total blood serum cholesterol levels of free-ranging meerkats have been reported as ranging from 3.55 to 11.1 mmol/L and consequently serve as a reference range for many insectivorous animal species.[24] In contrast, normal total blood serum cholesterol levels of domestic dogs are slightly higher, ranging from 7.5 to 20 mmol/L.[58]

Minerals

Minerals are reported as one of the most likely nutritional deficiencies of feeding insect-based diets.[3] Of particular concern are calcium and phosphorus. An inverse calcium:-phosphorus ratio (ie, < 1:1) due to insufficient dietary calcium, over-supplemented phosphorus, or insufficient dietary vitamin D_3 (or insufficient exposure to UVB lighting for reptiles) can all lead to hypocalcemia and secondary nutritional hyperparathyroidism (discussed in more detail in a later section).[59,60] Although dietary calcium must be ingested in equal to (1:1) or greater ($\geq$2:1) amounts than phosphorous to avoid calcium leaching from bones, most commercially raised insects have an inverse calcium:phosphorus ratio since they do not have a mineralized skeleton.[28,52] Those insect species with a mineralized exoskeleton generally includes the Dipterans, including houseflies and black soldier fly.[52] However, these species will also bioaccumulate other dietary minerals so a good understanding of the typical feeding program or typical mineral levels from those species is appropriate. Methods to increase mineral content of insects are discussed later in discussion, but gut loading and dusting may be effective at improving calcium:phosphorus ratios in deficient insects. For example, gut-loading locusts for 48 hours prior to feeding with 12.0% calcium (as-is), dusting of vitamins A and D_3 (see next section for details), and 10 hours per day of UVB exposure appeared to be the best combination to prevent metabolic bone disease in captive veiled chameleons (C calyptratus).[61]

Calcium requirements appear to be relatively low for tamanduas based on concentrations (DMB) of stomach contents of free-ranging specimens (0.11%) and dietary sources of wild termites (Nasutitermes spp., 0.26%).[62] Low calcium requirements may also be assumed for the giant anteater and hairy armadillo (Chaetophractus villosus) of which there are reports of hypercalcemia in captivity based on total blood calcium values above standard reference ranges for dogs (**Table 2**).[63] These values were suspected to be diet-induced and reportedly alleviated when the diet was changed, although dietary mineral data were not provided.[63,65] Comparatively, calcium requirements are likely greater for insectivorous reptiles and birds, particularly during times of egg laying. Maximum tolerable levels of dietary calcium and phosphorus have been reported for non-egg laying poultry (1.5% and 1.0%, respectively) and laying hens (5.0% and 0.8%, respectively), as well as recommended for reptiles (2.5% and 1.6%, respectively).[67,68] Much less is known about remaining mineral requirements for insectivores, and it is generally recommended to use the most similar domesticated animal model (or combination) as a guideline for dietary nutrient levels, in absence of specific knowledge of a need in a particular species.

Vitamins

Vitamin deficiencies are also not uncommon for animals fed insect-based diets.[3,69] Commercially raised insects for live feeding typically have low concentrations of vitamin A and vitamin D_3.[3,52] Recommended dietary provisions of vitamin D_3 have been reported for reptiles in general of 260 to 1800 IU/kg of diet with a maximum tolerable level of 5000 IU/kg of diet, and more specifically for carnivorous snakes of 500 to 1000 IU/kg of diet.[64,68,70] For the insectivorous veiled chameleon, dusting locusts immediately prior to feeding with 250,000 IU/kg vitamin A and 25,000 vitamin D_3, gut-loading with calcium (12% as-is), and 10 hours per day of UVB exposure appeared to be the best combination to prevent metabolic bone.[61]

Vitamin K deficiency has been documented in giant anteaters, although the provisioning of antibiotics may have been the basis for this pathology.[71] Antibiotics, via the modulation of gut microflora, have been shown to result in vitamin K deficiency.[72] Anteaters have also been reported to have a lower vitamin D requirement than strictly carnivorous mammals.[8] Anteaters and hairy armadillos have experienced hypervitaminosis D in captivity leading to hypercalcemia with reported Vitamin D levels (measured as serum 25(OH)D_3) above standard reference ranges for dogs and cats (see **Table 2**).[63] These values were suspected to be diet-induced and reportedly

Table 2
Total serum calcium (mmol/L), vitamin D (nmol/L), and diet and husbandry parameters of captive animal species with varying insectivorous tendencies and ranges of domestic dogs and cats commonly used for comparison

Species	Total Calcium[a,b]	Vitamin D[a,c]	Diet and Husbandry
Giant anteater[63]	3.7	808.7	Commercial insectivore pellet (gruel), insects
Giant anteater[63]	2.2	32.5	Gruel consisting of minced beef heart, fruit, commercial dog food, cooked oats, hard-boiled egg, dry cooked shrimp, water, honey, sieved peat, vitamin K supplement
Hairy armadillo[63]	2.7	379.4	Commercial insectivore pellet, insects, mincemeat, whole chick, hard-boiled egg
Hairy armadillo[63]	2.6	150.5	Insectivorous bird soft food mixed formula, miced beef meat, insects, whole chick, hard-boiled egg
Bearded dragon[64]		15.9 ± 3.6	Vitamin D_3 supplement (25%–400% of estimated daily requirement) via syringe, no UVB exposure
Bearded dragon[64]		198.5 ± 7.6	No vit D_3 supplement, UVB (295–300 nm) exposure (2–12 h/d)
Chinese water dragon[37]	9.4–16.0		Fed one of the 2 diets: (1) crickets, earthworms, superworms, waxworms, pinkie/fuzzy mouse, mineral supplement dusting, (2) commercial avian extruded pellet, crickets, and fruits
Veiled chameleon[61]	2.2	142	Locust nymphs without supplementation; UVB exposure
Veiled chameleon[61]	2.0	ND	Locust nymphs without supplementation; No UVB exposure
Veiled chameleon[61]	2.8	ND	Locust nymphs gut-loaded with calcium; UVB exposure
Veiled chameleon[61]	3.1	160	Locust nymphs gut-loaded with calcium; No UVB exposure
Veiled chameleon[61]	3.1	> 250	Locust nymphs gut-loaded with calcium, dusted with vitamin D_3; UVB exposure
Veiled chameleon	4.6	102	Locust nymphs gut-loaded with calcium, dusted and vitamin D_3; No UVB exposure
Domestic dog[63,65]	2.4 ± 0.18	17.2–139.9	–
Domestic cat[63,66]	2.25–2.83	59.0–2.06.6	–

Abbreviation: ND, not detectable.
[a] Blood serum.
[b] Liver.
[c] Measured as 25(OH)D_3.

alleviated when the diet was changed; however, no dietary vitamin data were provided.[63] Furthermore, tamanduas were reported to have hypercalcemia due to hypervitaminosis D and A when fed diets containing 3200 to 6300 IU/kg vitamin D_2 although blood serum values were not reported.[63] Insects are generally a poor source of vitamin A and a much more likely source of dietary carotenoids.[52] While some insectivores are able to convert ß-carotene to vitamin A, dietary vitamin A is still recommended for all species.[73]

Unfortunately, measuring vitamin A status is difficult. Serum retinol is not reflective of total body vitamin A. Liver retinol is a more accurate indicator, although unlikely to be an appropriate method of assessing vitamin A status in captively managed exotic animals. In dogs fed high levels of vitamin A, serum retinol was unchanged, although serum retinyl esters did increase with increasing dietary vitamin A.[74] Maximum tolerable levels of dietary vitamin A (IU/kg of diet) have been determined for domestic dogs (33,330) and cats (100,000), growing chickens (15,000), and egg-laying chickens (40,000).[67] Of these model species, a maximum tolerable level of dietary vitamin D_3 has only been determined for growing chickens at 40,000 IU/kg of diet.[67]

NUTRITIONAL COMPOSITION OF INSECTS

Over the past several years there has been increased attention regarding the nutritional composition of insect species as their use has expanded from primarily live feeding applications to dry ingredients in pelleted and extruded diets. Insects can provide high quality nutritional value as well as higher edible fractions than traditional animal proteins.[50] Insects are a good source of protein, fat, and carbohydrates, and thus energy, but the ratio of these nutrients can be dependent upon the insect's developmental pattern.

There are three types of development that insects can experience: ametaboly, hemimetaboly, and holometaboly.[7] Ametaboly is essentially a lack of defined developmental stages where the insect hatches from the egg in a form nearly identical to the adult, but is not yet reproductively mature.[7] Hemimetaboly is the process of incomplete metamorphosis where the insect hatches in an immature form and goes through developmental stages to become the mature form.[7,51] Holometaboly is the process of complete metamorphosis where the insect hatches in a larval form and develops through several stages that lead to pupation and emergence as a mature adult of a completely different form (ie, larvae to adult fly).[7,51] The nutrient composition (ranges when possible) of four common feeder insect species is presented in **Table 3**.

Protein and Carbohydrates

Insects are generally a good source of protein and amino acids. Protein composition of commercially raised insects is reported to vary between 20% and 80%.[51] An average of 55% crude protein (DMB) has been reported across free ranging insects representing 13 insect orders known to be commonly ingested by insectivorous primates.[7] All essential amino acids are typically present and make up 46% to 96% of insect protein content.[7,76] Total protein content and amino acid concentrations can vary throughout an insect's life cycle and may be affected by the metamorphosis process of the insect, either not present (ametabolous), incomplete (hemimetabolous), or complete (holometabolous).[7,51] In house crickets (*Acheta domesticus*), a hemimetabolous species, protein content is relatively consistent across life stages.[51] In contrast, protein content of black soldier fly (*Hermetia illucens*) larvae, a holometabolous species, is more variable as a result of increased fat content as the larvae ages in preparation for complete metamorphosis.[50,51] Methionine and cystine are typically the first-limiting amino acids in most insect-based diets.[50,51] Protein digestibility of different insect species and forms has been most studied in poultry and rats of which results have been comparable or just slightly lower than the benchmark of milk protein casein.[51]

Although free-ranging insects typically contain low levels of non-structural carbohydrates (NSC; starches, sugars, and other oligosaccharides), a recent review of published data demonstrated NSC to make up 5.0% to 51.6% of the nutritional composition across 16 free-ranging insect species representing five orders [7,78]; however, the NSC contents may be due to gut fill, although this was not discussed. In another comparison of nutritional composition of insects, soluble carbohydrates were much lower in mealworms (*Tenebrio molitor*) and crickets (species not identified) at 3.0% and 6.0% (DMB, respectively) compared to honeypot ants (*Myrmecocytus melliger*) at 81% (DMB).[7] This difference was assumed to be due to natural behaviors of honeypot ants to gorge themselves, which may also be the case in some of the higher NSC contents reported in other species.[7] This demonstrates the potential benefits of appropriately gut-loading insects prior to feeding insectivorous animals.

Insects are also composed of structural carbohydrates. Crude fiber has been reported in 51 free-ranging insect species representing six orders, ranging from 1.0% to 28.1% (DMB).[78] Chitin, a structural polymer found in the cuticle of insects and crustaceans, is considered to act similarly to structural carbohydrates within the vertebrate gastrointestinal tract. Chitin can comprise up to 60% (DMB) of insect weight, depending on species.[79] Recent literature reports several functional benefits of chitin including as an antimicrobial and prebiotic, in addition to being a source of nitrogen and energy as described above.[80]

Lipids

Fat composition of insects can vary widely from less than 10% to 70% (DMB) and can be affected by the insect's diet, life stage, and rearing conditions.[51,55] Average fat content of free-ranging adult life stage insects across 13 orders has been reported at 20.7% (DMB).[7] Much like protein content, fat content is also affected by an insect's metamorphosis process with fat content increasing as larvae age in holometabolous species, since they utilize that lipid to fuel the process of metamorphosis.[50] Crude fat content of commercially raised insects is typically higher than free-ranging insects but lower in linoleic acid, an essential fatty acid for all mammals studied to date.[51] Commercially raised larvae of the black soldier fly are unique compared to other insect species as their fat content is naturally high in the saturated fatty acid, lauric acid, regardless of diet.[50,51] This medium-chain fatty acid hosts antimicrobial functions against gram-positive pathogens, an ability to regulate total cholesterol levels, and a faster energy source.[50,81]

Minerals

Most commercially reared insects are deficient in calcium resulting in an inverse calcium:phosphorus ratio. Recent reviews have reported similar calcium concentrations of crickets and mealworms to average 0.10% (DMB).[50,80] An exception is larvae of the black soldier fly which accumulate dietary calcium in their exoskeleton resulting in a positive calcium:phosphorus ratio averaging 2:1.[46,50,51] However, these species will also bioaccumulate other dietary minerals so a good understanding of the typical feeding program or mineral levels from those species is appropriate. Other than calcium, electrolytes (Mg, Na, K) and microminerals (Zn, Cu, Fe, Mn) are generally found in adequate amounts to meet the known nutrient requirements of birds, fish, and mammals.[52]

Table 3
Nutritional composition (as-is basis, ranges presented when possible) of commercially raised insect species commonly used for feeding captive insectivorous animals

Nutrient	Black Soldier Fly Larvae (Hermetia illucens)	Cricket (Adults, Acheta domesticus)	Mealworm (Tenbrio molitor)	Superworm (Zophobas morio)
Moisture, %[50,75]	61.2	69.2–72.5	61.9–68.9	42.1–63.0
Crude protein, %[50,75]	17.5	16.5–20.5	18.7	18.6–19.7
Arginine, %[50]	1.23	1.25	0.97	0.96
Histidine, %[50]	0.59	0.48	0.59	0.60
Isoleucine, %[50]	0.76	0.94	0.94	0.93
Leucine, %[50]	1.21	2.05	1.99	1.91
Lysine, %[50]	1.19	1.10	1.19	1.03
Methionine, %[50]	0.34	0.30	0.24	0.21
Methionine + Cystine, %[50]	0.44	0.47	0.40	0.36
Phenylalanine, %[50]	0.76	0.65	0.66	0.68
Threonine, %[50]	0.68	0.74	0.77	0.78
Tryptophan, %[50]	0.30	0.13	0.15	0.18
Valine, %[50]	1.29	1.07	1.10	1.03
Crude fat, %[50,55]	9.8–14.0	6.8	9.7–13.4	17.7–25.2
Saturated fat, %[55,76,77]	6.9	2.5	2.8	7.2
Monounsaturated fat, %[55,76,77]	1.5	1.3	4.7	5.3
Polyunsaturated fat, %[55,76,77]	1.2	0.5	2.1	3.8
Total omega-6, %[55,76]	1.0	0.4	2.3	
Total omega-3, %[55,76]	0.2	0.02	0.3	
NFE, %[50]	0.8	0.0	2.7	1.1
ADF, %[50,75]	0.3	1.8–3.2	2.2–2.5	2.3–2.7
Chitin, %[50]	2.5	2.1	ND	ND
Ash, %[50]	3.5	1.1	0.9	1.0

Ca:P	2.6:1	0.13:1–0.75:1	0.07:1	0.1:1
Calcium, %[50,75]	0.93	0.03–0.04	0.02	0.02–0.03
Phosphorus, %[50,75]	0.36	0.22–0.30	0.26–0.29	0.21–0.24
Magnesium, %[50,75]	0.17	0.02–0.03	0.06–0.08	0.04–0.05
Sodium, %[50,75]	0.09	0.11–0.13	0.02–0.05	0.04–0.05
Potassium, %[50,75]	0.45	0.29–0.35	0.34	0.29–0.32
Chloride, %[50,75]	0.12	0.22–0.23	0.18–0.19	0.15–0.16
Copper, ppm[50,75]	4.0	6.2–6.3	6.1–8.3	3.6
Iron, ppm[50,75]	66.6	17.5–19.3	20.6–20.7	16.5–19.9
Manganese, ppm[50,75]	61.8	8.7–11.5	3.2–5.2	3.7–4.3
Zinc, ppm[50,75]	56.2	54.3–67.1	49.5–52.0	30.2–30.7
Vitamin A[a], IU/kg[50,75]	< 1000	< 1000	< 1000	< 1000
Vitamin D3, IU/kg[50]	< 251	< 251	< 251	< 251
Vitamin E, IU/kg[50,75]	9.2	19.7–53.7	< 36.2	7.7–163
Thiamin, ppm[50]	7.7	0.4	2.4	0.6
Riboflavin, ppm[50]	16.2	34.1	8.1	7.5
Pantothenic acid, ppm[50]	38.5	23.0	26.2	19.4
Niacin, ppm[50]	71.0	38.4	40.7	32.3
Pyridoxine, ppm[50]	6.0	2.3	8.1	3.2
Folic acid, ppm[50]	2.7	1.5	1.6	0.7

Abbreviation: ND, not detectable.
[a] From retinol.

Vitamins

Many commercially raised insect species are an inadequate source of preformed vitamin A, vitamin D_3, and vitamin E.[3,52,61] Although insects can synthesize dietary carotenoids into retinal, this process takes place in structures of compound eyes which are lacking in larval life stages of insects.[52] Gut-loading with retinol is often not successful, although gut-loading of insects with carotenoids has been demonstrated to be successful.[82]

Vitamin D_3 levels are generally low in insects. Some insects, such as house crickets, have the ability to convert provitamin-D_3 (7-dehydrocholesterol) into vitamin D_3 if provided sufficient exposure to full spectrum UVB lighting.[52] However, crickets still contain minimal vitamin D_3 levels compared to minimum dietary vitamin D recommendations for domestic dogs and cats of 500 IU/kg of diet.[54] It is generally recommended that vitamin D_3 nutrition be accomplished via other means, primarily through dietary supplementation and exposure to ultraviolet light.[52] Vitamin E can be accumulated by most commercially raised insects from dietary sources, and thus may vary by supplier.[50] The B-vitamin content of insects, at least that of commercial feeder insects, appears to be adequate to meet nutrient requirements, with the exception of thiamine for which variable levels have been found in commercial feeder insects, and vitamin C which can vary significantly as well.[83,84]

RECOMMENDATIONS FOR FEEDING INSECTIVORES
Diet Item Considerations

As previously mentioned, insectivorous animals require nutrients rather than specific food items. However, provisioning diet items that allow for natural behaviors for foraging and food processing may have benefits well beyond that of essential nutrition. As previously mentioned, insectivores in free-ranging habitats consume a wide variety of insect species, and this diversity and variety is generally not available in captively managed settings. Thus, commercially reared feeder insects often supply any insect-derived dietary component, and other food items are offered to complement the insect-based nutrition and meet other requirements (both nutritionally and behaviorally) that the animal may have. In addition to the consideration of the physical form of the diet offered, the method of provisioning should be considered as well. For animals that would normally catch moving prey, live feeder insects may be preferable to dry diet items. For animals that would normally source insects from within some substrate (eg, through tree bark, within a termite mound, and so forth), simulation of this foraging behavior and the use of appropriately sized food items may promote more natural behaviors.

Common food items fed to captive insectivores include insects, insectivore pellets, chicken eggs, whole chicks, mice, beef, commercial dog food, commercial cat food, fruits, vegetables, rice, and mineral and vitamin supplements.[11,12,85] Proximate nutrients for common invertebrate prey, whole vertebrate prey, raw meat diets, and commercial diets fed to captive insectivorous animals are reported in **Table 4**. Obviously, there are a large number of commercial cat and dog diets that may be used in zoos and aquaria, and for which nutrient concentrations should be considered similarly.

As previously mentioned, commercial feeder insects may be deficient in certain essential nutrients. Methods to increase targeted nutrient content of insects include gut loading and dusting. Gut-loading of insects involves provisioning them diets that contain high levels of the nutrient of concern (eg, calcium) for some period of time, during which the insect gut becomes enriched in that nutrient. The insect can be fed the gut-loading diet for approximately 24 to 72 hours before being offered to an animal.[52] Nutrient concentrations are enhanced by being present as ingested feed in the gastrointestinal tract of the insect.[52] Nutrients for which gut-loading has proven successful include calcium, polyunsaturated fatty acids, carotenoids, vitamin D_3, and vitamin E.[52,91]

Dusting involves the application of nutrient-rich powder to the exoskeleton of insects and is most effective with insects that cannot groom themselves. Thus, it is important to dust insects immediately prior to offering them as a food item. Dusting has been proven successful to increase calcium and vitamin A content.[52]

Finally, when feeding a diet consisting of multiple food items, it is important to be aware of food item sorting behaviors. In a reported case study of four lesser hedgehogs with metabolic bone disease, it was determined that at least two of the animals selectively ate only the insects which were un-supplemented, and likely lead to phosphorus deficiency from inadequate dietary vitamin D.[92]

CONTROVERSIES
Obesity

Captively managed animals are often over-conditioned, and insectivorous species are no exception. This may be due to inappropriate diet components (eg, excessively fatty diets rich in larval stage insects) and to providing excess calories relative to the animal's

Table 4
Average proximate nutrient composition on a dry matter basis (except dry matter) of common invertebrate prey, whole prey items, raw meat diets, and commercial diets fed to captive insectivores

Item	Dry Matter, %	Crude Protein, %	Crude Fat, %	Ash, %	Gross Energy, Kcal/g
Invertebrate Prey[50]					
Cricket (adult, *Acheta domesticus*)	30.8	66.6	22.1	3.6	NR
Mealworm (*Tenebrio molitor*)	38.1	62.1	44.5	3.0	NR
Black soldier fly larvae (*Hermetia illucens*)	38.8	45.1	36.1	9.0	NR
Whole Vertebrate Prey[86]					
Mouse (domestic), neonate (<3g)	18.2	44.2	30.1	8.5	6.65
Mouse (domestic), juvenile (3–10g)	32.7	55.8	23.6	11.8	5.25
Rat, neonate (<10g)	20.8	57.9	23.7	12.2	5.30
Rat, juvenile (10–50g)	30.0	56.1	27.5	14.8	5.55
Rat, adult (>50g)	33.9	61.8	32.6	9.8	6.37
Chick, hatchling (1-day-old)	25.6	64.9	22.4	6.4	5.80
Raw Meat Diets[87]					
Beef-based	34.9	52.4	33.1	NR	6.3
Horse-based	36.9	50.3	31.6	NR	6.1
Pork-based	33.0	51.0	39.9	NR	6.7
Commercial Extruded Diets[88–90]					
Exotic Feline diet	88%	40.9	22.7	9.7	NR
Exotic Canine diet	88%	33.0	20.5	10.0	NR
Insectivore diet	88%	33.0	12.5	8.9	NR

Abbreviation: NR, not reported.

activity level and metabolic needs. Diets are often provided in one or two meals in comparison to regular foraging or hunting behaviors in captive counterparts, and acquisition of the diet requires very little energy expenditure on the animal's part.[93] Over-conditioned animals are at risk for several secondary issues such as reproductive difficulties, skeletal abnormalities, and dental disease.[93,94] An additional difficulty resulting from over-conditioned animals is proper anaesthetization which is often required for examinations of animals housed in zoos or aquaria.[95] The most common recommendations for weight loss are to reduce energy-dense foods and increase activity.[96] A recommendation for combatting obesity in captive Chinese pangolins is the addition of 5.0% ground chitin to the diet as this may slightly decrease dry matter, energy, and protein digestibility while promoting improved fecal consistency.[9,23]

Hypercholesterolemia

Hypercholesterolemia is a metabolic disorder characterized by high blood serum cholesterol and high low-density lipoproteins (LDL).[97] High blood serum cholesterol of meerkats has been reported as a consequence of high dietary cholesterol, which can lead to meningeal cholesterol granulomas.[24] Cholesterol is present in higher concentrations in vertebrate-based diets compared to invertebrate-based diets (since insects cannot synthesize cholesterol), and captive insectivores may still be fed diets high in vertebrate-based food items. As previously mentioned, blood serum cholesterol levels of free-ranging meerkats have been reported as 3.55 to 11.1 mmol/L and consequently used as a reference range.[24] A recent study investigating cholesterol levels of 11 captive male slender-tailed meerkats (*Suricata suricatta*) demonstrated that animals fed a primarily vertebrate-based diet (containing whole mice or chicks) had cholesterol levels indicative of hypercholesteremia (ranging from 11.1 to 23.5 mmol/L, mean 15.6 ± 3.94). When those animals were transitioned to a diet containing lower levels of the vertebrate prey items, serum cholesterol levels declined significantly after 8 months ($P < .05$, 3.6–9.7 mmol/L, mean 6.77 ± 1.53).[24]

Metabolic Bone Disease

Metabolic bone disease (MBD) has been reported in several captive insectivorous species such as lesser hedgehogs (*Echinops telfairi*), bearded dragons (*Pogona vitticeps*), and veiled chameleons (*Chamaeleo calyptratus*).[61,92,98] This disease is a general term for a collection of issues often characterized by poor bone mineralization, skeletal deformities, tetany, and weakness, all of which may lead to fractures.[3,60,61] Metabolic bone disease has been linked to vitamin A deficiency, vitamin D_3 deficiency, and calcium deficiency.[60,61,92] Vitamin A deficiency can be a result of feeding diets with high amounts of vertebrate meat and has also been associated with further consequences including eye, skin, respiratory, and neurologic diseases, particularly in reptiles.[61,96] Calcium and vitamin D_3 deficiencies are often the result of inadequately supplemented insects in the diet or inadequate UVB exposure for reptiles.[96] Diets based primarily on vertebrate meat and insufficiently supplemented is also a likely cause of calcium deficiency.[54]

Treatment of MBD is dependent upon the cause although adjusting calcium, vitamins A and D_3, and UVB exposure are common remedies. For reptiles with a suspected calcium deficiency, addition of calcium carbonate as 1.5% of the diet (DMB) has been recommended to help reverse MBD.[96] This is in addition to ensuring unhindered access to full-spectrum UVB lighting.[96] Gut-loading locusts for 48 hours prior to feeding with 12.0% calcium (as-is), dusting of vitamins A and D_3, and 10 hours per day of UVB exposure appeared to be the best combination to prevent metabolic bone disease in captive veiled chameleons (*C calyptratus*).[61]

Nutritional Secondary Hyperparathyroidism

Nutritional secondary hyperparathyroidism (NSHP) is a specific type of MBD where the parathyroid gland over-secretes parathormone, a hormone that helps regulate calcium and phosphorus levels in the intestines (calcium absorption), kidneys (resorption of calcium), and bones (calcium release).[99–101] Parathormone over-secretion occurs when blood calcium is low, often caused by inadequate dietary calcium or vitamin D_3 (as vitamin D mediates this process).[99,100,102] Symptoms of NSHP include skeletal deformities (due to release of calcium from bone) that may or may not be apparent in early stages of the disease.[99] Animals with NSHP often have difficulty holding their head up fully or putting their full weight onto their limbs.[102] Treatment should include balancing the diet for adequate calcium and a positive calcium:phosphorus ratio ($\geq$2:1), and adequate vitamin D_3. Restoration of parathyroid gland function is assumed to take 6 to 12 weeks based on when clinical improvements are most often identified.[102]

DISCUSSION

Outside of captivity, there is an overwhelming diversity of insects consumed by insectivorous animals. This diversity is a result of seasonal, temporal, and insect life stages, among other factors, that are not easily mimicked in captivity. In general, free-ranging insectivores have lower BMRs than strictly carnivorous species, indicating the heavy body condition of many captive insectivores is likely due to higher dietary energy provisions than necessary.[43] This may be partly due to feeding insectivores diets primarily based on vertebrate items that are high in fat, and therefore, energy dense. Feeding insectivores primarily vertebrate-based meat with insufficient mineral supplementation can also lead to calcium deficiency.[54] With calcium deficiency also being a concern when feeding insects as food items, there is a need for veterinary and nutrition professionals to critically analyze dietary mineral provisions and mineral balance of insectivore diets. Fat soluble vitamins A and D should also be of primary concern when developing diets and feeding protocols for insectivores, as commercially raised insects are poor sources of these important nutrients.

SUMMARY

Although insectivores are present across nearly all taxa, much less is known about their nutritional requirements compared to species of other dietary strategies, such as carnivores and herbivores. Therefore, nutrient recommendations have not been fully developed and are based heavily on established requirements of species with similar digestive tract morphology and physiology. Additionally, insectivorous animals have unique adaptations for apprehending and consuming insects that should be acknowledged as part of their captive dietary management. Insectivore diets should include insect components with known nutritional composition that are complemented with other available feed items to provide a complete diet.

CLINICS CARE POINTS

- Veterinary and nutrition professionals should emphasize the importance of balancing dietary micronutrients for insectivores, particularly calcium, phosphorus, and vitamins A and D_3 (with the addition of UVB exposure for reptiles).
- An aim of insectivore diets should include minimizing energy-dense vertebrate-based prey that may over-supply saturated fats and cholesterol, and under-supply calcium.

- Species-specific adaptations for the apprehension and consumption of insects should be considered when developing and providing diets for insectivores.

DISCLOSURE

The authors have no conflicts of interest.

REFERENCES

1. Vafidis J, Smith J, Thomas R. Climate change and insectivore ecology, eLS. Chichester: John Wiley & Sons Ltd; 2019. p. 1–8.
2. D'Agostino J. Insectivores (insectivora, macroscelidea, scandentia). In: Miller RE, Fowler ME, editors. Fowler's zoo and wild animal medicine8. St. Louis: Elsevier; 2015. p. 275–81.
3. Ferrie GM, Alford VC, Atkinson J, et al. Nutrition and health in amphibian husbandry. Zoo Biol 2014;33(6):485–501.
4. Nyffeler M, Şekercioğlu CH, Whelan CJ. Insectivorous birds consume an estimated 400-500 million tons of prey annually. Sci Nat 2018;105(47).
5. Stevens CE, Hume ID. Contributions of microbes in vertebrate gastrointestinal tract to production and conservation of nutrients. Physiol Rev 1998;78(2): 393–427.
6. Gallo JA, Abba AM, Elizalde L, et al. First study on food habits of anteaters, Myrmecophaga tridactyla and Tamandua tetradactyla, at the southern limit of their distribution. Mammalia 2017;81(6).
7. Rothman JM, Raubenheimer D, Bryer MAH, et al. Nutritional contributions of insects to primate diets: implications for primate evolution. J Human Evol 2014;71:59–69.
8. Gull JM, Stahl M, Osmann C, et al. Digestive physiology of captive giant anteaters (Myrmecophaga tridactyla): Determinants of faecal dry matter content. J Anim Physiol Anim Nutr 2015;99:565–76.
9. Lin MF, Chang C-Y, Yang CW, et al. Aspects of digestive anatomy, feed intake and digestion in the Chinese pangolin (Manis pentadactyla) at Taipei Zoo. Zoo Biol 2015;9999:1–9.
10. Tucker AS. Salivary gland adaptations: modification of the glands for novel uses. In: Tucker AS, Miletech I, editors. Frontiers of oral biology. Salivary glands: development, adaptations and disease14. Basel: Kargel; 2010. p. 21–31.
11. Clark A, Silva-Fletcher A, Fox M, et al. Survey of feeding practices, body condition and faeces consistency in captive ant-eating mammals in the UK. J Zoo Aquar Res 2016;4(4):183–95.
12. Ma J-E, Li L-M, Jiang H-Y, et al. Acidic mammalian chitinase gene is highly expressed in the special oxyntic glands of Manis javanica. FEBS Open Bio 2018;1247–55.
13. Modrackova N, Stovicek A, Burtscher J, et al. The bifidobacterial distribution in the microbiome of captive primates reflects parvorder and feed specialization of the host. Sci Rep 2021;11:15273.
14. Taniguchi M, Nambu M, Katakura Y, et al. Adhesion mechanisms of Bifidobacterium animals subsp. Lactis JCM 10602 to dietary fiber. Biosci Microbiota Food Health 2021;40(1):59–64.
15. Stull VJ, Finer E, Bergmans RS, et al. Impact of edible cricket consumption on gut microbiota in healthy adults, a double-blind, randomized crossover trial. Sci Rep 2018;8:10762.

16. Ashwell KWS. Development of the olfactory pathways in platypus and echidna. Brain Behav Evol 2012;79(1):45–56.

17. Jones G, Teeling EC. The evolution of echolocation in bats. Trends Ecol Evol 2006;21(3):149–56.

18. Czech-Damal NU, Dehnhardt G, Manger P, et al. Passive electroreception in aquatic mammals. J Comp Physiol 2013;199:555–63.

19. Manger PR, Collins R, Pettigrew JD. Histological observations on presumed electroreceptors and mechanoreceptors in the beak skin of the long-beaked echidna, Zaglossus bruijnii. Proc R Soc London, B 1997;264:165–72.

20. Catania KC. Evolution of sensory specializations in insectivores. Anat Rec 2005;1038–50.

21. Marasco PD, Tsuruda PR, Bautista DM, et al. Fine structure of Eimer's organ in the coast mole (Scapanus orarius). Anatom Rec 2007;290:437–48.

22. Doolan SP, Macdonald DW. Diet and foraging behavior of group-living meerkats, Suricata suricatta, in the southern Kalahari. J Zool 1996;239(4):697–716.

23. Wang X-M, Janssens GPJ, Xie C-G, et al. To save pangolins: a nutritional perspective. Animals 2022;12:3137.

24. Dobbs P, Liptovszky M, Moittie S. Dietary management of hypercholesterolemia in a bachelor group of zoo-housed slender-tailed meerkats Suricata suricatta. J Zoo Aqua Res 2020;8(4):294–6.

25. Morford S, Meyers MA. Giant anteater (Myrmecophaga tridactyla) diet survey. Edentata 2003;5:20–4.

26. Toledo N, Bargo MS, Vizcaíno SF, et al. Evolution of body size in anteaters and sloths (Xenartha, Pilosa): phylogeny, metabolism, diet and substrate preferences. Earth Environ Sci Trans R Soc Edinb 2015;106(4):289–301.

27. Stone ZL, Tasker E, Maron M. Patterns of invertebrate food availability and the persistence of an avian insectivore on the brink. Austral Ecol 2020;44(4):680–90.

28. Razeng E, Watson DM. Nutritional composition of the preferred prey of insectivorous birds: popularity reflects quality. J Avian Biol 2015;46:89–96.

29. Smithsonian's National Zoo. Animals. Smithsonian's National Zoo and Conservation Biology Institute. n.d. Available at https://nationalzoo.si.edu/animals. Accessed May 1, 2023.

30. San Diego Zoo. Wildlife. San Diego Zoo Wildlife Alliance. n.d. Available at https://zoo.sandiegozoo.org/wildlife. Accessed May 1, 2023.

31. Detroit Zoo. Zoo animals. n.d. Available at https://detroitzoo.org/animals/zoo-animals/. Accessed May 1, 2023.

32. Brevard Zoo. Meet the animals. n.d. Available at https://brevardzoo.org/animal-wellness/?to=animals. Accessed May 1, 2023.

33. Rodríguez A, Negro JJ, Bustamante J, et al. Establishing a lesser kestrel colony in an urban environment for research purposes. J Raptor Res 2013;47(2):214–8.

34. Los Angeles Zoo. Our animals. n.d. Available at https://lazoo.org/explore-your-zoo/our-animals/. Accessed May 1, 2023.

35. Elston JJ, Carney J, Quinones G, et al. Use of novel nest boxes by carmine bee-eaters (Merops nubicus) in captivity. Zoo Biol 2007;26:27–39.

36. Ramirez AA, Perez K, Telemeco RS. Thermoregulation and thermal performance of crested geckos (Correlophus ciliatus) suggest an extended optimality hypothesis for the evolution of thermoregulatory set-points. J Exp Zool 2021;335:86–95.

37. Mayer J, Knoll J, Innis C, et al. Characterizing the hematologic and plasma chemistry profiles of captive Chinese water dragons, Physignathus oncincinus. J Herpetol Med Surg 2005;15(3):16–23.

38. Melero A, Novellas R, Mollol C, et al. Ultrasonographic appearance of the coelomic cavity organs in healthy veiled chameleons (Chamaeleo calyptratus) and panther chameleons (Furcifer pardalis). Vet Radiol Ultrasound 2020;61: 58–66.

39. Hagey TJ, Losos JB, Harmon LJ. Cruise foraging of invasive chameleon (Chamaeleo jacksonii xantholophus) in Hawai'i. Brevoria 2010;519(1):1–7.

40. Villamar-Duque TE, Cruz-Elizalde R, Ramírez-Bautista A. Reproduction of the Bromeliad arboreal alligator lizard, Abronia taeniata (Squamata: Anguidae), in a temperate environment of central Mexico. Salamandra 2019;55(4):221–30.

41. Kaiser K, Devito J, Jones CG, et al. Effects of anthropogenic noise on endocrine and reproductive function in White's treefrog, Litoria caerulea. Conserv Physiol 2015;3:1–8.

42. Denver Zoo. Animals. n.d. Available at https://denverzoo.org/animals/. Accessed May 1, 2023.

43. Nagy KA, Girard IA. Brown TK. Energetics of free-ranging mammals, reptiles, and birds. Annu Rev Nutr 1999;19:247–77.

44. Nagy KA. Food requirements of wild animals: predictive equations for free-living mammals, reptiles, and birds. Nutr Abstr Rev 2001;B71:21R–31R.

45. National Research Council (NRC). Nutrient requirements of dogs and cats. Washinton, D.C: The National Academies Press; 2006.

46. Finke MD. Estimate of chitin in raw whole insects. Zoo Biol 2007;26:105–15.

47. Zárate V, Mufari JR, Abalos Luna LG, et al. Assessment of feeding behavior of the zoo-housed lesser anteater (Tamandua tetradactyla) and nutritional values of natural prey. J Zool Botan Gard 2022;3:19–31.

48. Tabata E, Kashimura A, Uehara M, et al. High expression of acidic chitinase and chitin digestibility in the stomach of common marmoset (Callithrix jacchus), an insectivorous nonhuman primate. Sci Rep 2019;9:159.

49. Leuchner L, Nofs SA, Dierenfeld ES, et al. Chitin supplementation in the diets of captive giant anteaters (Myrmecophaga tridactyla) for improved gastrointestinal function. J Zoo Aquar Res 2017;5(2):92–6.

50. Koutsos L, McComb A, Finke M. Insect composition and uses in animal feeding applications: a brief review. Ann Entomol Soc Am 2019;112(6):544–51.

51. Oonincx DGAB, Finke MD. Nutritional value of insects and ways to manipulate their composition. J Insects Food and Feed 2021;7(5):639–59.

52. Oonincx DGAB, Finke MD. Insects as a complete nutritional source. J Insects Feed Food 2023;9(5):541–3.

53. Nofs SA, Dierenfeld ES, Backus RC. Effect of increasing taurine and methionine supplementation on urinary taurine excretion in a model insectivore, the giant anteater (Myrmecophaga tridactyla). J Anim Physiol Anim Nutr 2018;102: e316–25.

54. Lewis LD, Morris ML, Hand MS. Nutrients. In Small animal clinical nutrition III. 3rd edition. Topeka: Mark Morris Associates; 1997. p. 1–24.

55. Benzertiha A, Kierończyk B, Rawski M, et al. Insect fat in animal nutrition – a review. Sciendo 2020;20(4):1217–40.

56. Shipley JR, Twining CW, Mathieu-Resuge M, et al. Climate change shifts the timing of nutritional flux from aquatic insects. Curr Biol 2022;32:1342–9.

57. Haas E, Kim Y, Stanley D. Why can insects not biosynthesize cholesterol? Insect Biochem Physiol 2023;112(3):e21983.

58. Borin-Crivellenti S, Crivellenti LZ, de Oliveira FR, et al. Effect of phytosterols on reducing low-density lipoprotein cholesterol in dogs. Dom Anim Endocrin 2021; 76:106610.

59. Boykin KL, Carter RT, Butler-Perez K, et al. Digestibility of black soldier fly larvae (Hermetia illucens) fed to leopard geckos (Eublepharis macularius). PONE 2020;15(5):e0232496.
60. Dierenfeld ES, King J. Digestibility and mineral availability of Phoenix worms, Hermetia illucens, ingested by mountain chicken frogs, Leptodactylus fallax. J Herp Med Surg 2008;18(3/4):100–5.
61. Hoby S, Wenker C, Robert N, et al. Nutritional metabolic bone disease in juvenile veiled chameleons (Chamaeleo calyptratus) and its prevention. J Nutr 2010; 140(11):1923–31.
62. Oyarzun SE, Crawshaw GJ, Valdes EV. Nutrition of the tamandua: I. Nutrient composition of termites (Nasutitermes spp.) and stomach contents from wild tamanduas (Tamandua tetradactyla). Zoo Biol 1996;15:509–24.
63. Cole GC, Naylor AD, Hurst E, et al. Hypervitaminosis D in a giant anteater (Myrmecophaga tridactyla) and a large hairy armadillo (Chaetophractus villosus) receiving a commercial insectivore diet. J Zoo Wildl Med 2020;51(1):245–8.
64. Oonincx DGAB, Stevens Y, van den Borne JJGC, et al. Effects of vitamin D3 supplementation and UVB exposure on the growth and plasma concentration of vitamin D3 metabolites in juvenile bearded dragons. Comp Biochem Physiol B 2010;156:122–8.
65. Szenci O, Felkai F. Märcz, I, Takács E. Ionized calcium, total calcium and acid-base values of blood in healthy and acidotic dogs. J Vet Med Sci 1988;35(1–10): 125–8.
66. Cornell University, College of Veterinary Medicine. Animal Health Diagnostic Center. 2017. Available at: https://www.vet.cornell.edu/animal-health-diagnostic-center/laboratories/clinical-pathology/reference-intervals/chemistry. Accessed May 26, 2023.
67. National Research Council (NRC). Mineral tolerance of animals, 2nd revised edition. Washington, D.C: National Academies Press; 2005. p. 496.
68. Donoghue S, McKeown S. Nutrition of captive reptiles. In: Rupley AE, Jenkins JR, editors. Veterinary clinics of North America: exotic animal practice, 2nd edition (Husbandry and Nutrition1. Los Osos, California: Diamond Head Publishing; 1999. p. 69–91.
69. Michaels CJ, Ferguson A, Newton-Youens J, et al. Effects of sex and whole life cycle UVB irradiation on performance and mineral and vitamin D3 contents in feeder crickets. J Zool Bot Gard 2022;3:488–98.
70. Allen ME, Oftedal OT. The nutrition of carnivorous reptiles. In: Murphy JB, Adler K, Collins JT, editors. Captive management and conservation of amphibians and reptiles. New York: Society for the Study of Amphibians and Reptiles; 1994. p. 71–82.
71. Valdes EV, Brenes Soto A. Feeding and nutrition of anteaters. In: Miller RE, Fowler M, editors. Fowler's zoo and wild animal medicine: Current therapy7. St. Louis: Elsevier Saunders; 2012. p. 378–83.
72. Shirakawa H, Komai M, Kimura S. Antibiotic-induced vitamin K deficiency and the role of the presence of intestinal flora. Int J Vitam Nutr Res 1990;60(3): 245–51.
73. Freel T, Koutsos E, Minter LJ, et al. Cane toad (Rhinella marina) vitamin A, vitamin E, and carotenoid kinetics. Zoo Biol 2022;41(1):34–43.
74. Morris PJ, Salt C, Raila J, et al. Safety evaluation of vitamin A in growing dogs. Br J Nutr 2012;108(10):1800–9.
75. Finke MD. Complete nutrient content of four species of commercially available feeder insects fed enhanced diets during growth. Zoo Biol 2015;34:554–64.

76. Udomsil N, Imsoonthornruksa S, Gosalawit C, et al. Nutritional values and functional properties of house cricket (Acheta domesticus) and field cricket (Gryllus bimaculatus). Food Sci Technol Res 2019;25(4):597–605.

77. Adámková A, Kouřimská L, Borkovcová M, et al. Nutritional values of edible Coleoptera (Tenebrio molitor, Zophobas Morio and Alphitobius diaperinus) reared in the Czech Republic. Potr Sci J Food Indust 2016;10(1):663–71.

78. Hlongwane ZT, Slotow R, Munyai TC. Nutritional composition of edible insects consumed in Africa: a systematic review. Nutrients 2020;12:2786.

79. Koutsos E, Modica B, Freel T. Immunomodulatory potential of black soldier fly larvae: applications beyond nutrition in animal feeding programs. Transl Anim Sci 2022;6:1–9.

80. Hahn T, Roth A, Febel E, et al. New methods for high-accuracy insect chitin measurement. J Sci Food Agric 2018;98:5069–73.

81. Valdés F, Villanueva V, Durán E, et al. Insects as feed for companion and exotic pets: a current trend. Animals 2022;12:1450.

82. Ogilvy V, Preziosi RF, Fidgett AL. A brighter future for frogs? The influence of carotenoids on the health, development and reproductive success of the red-eye tree frog. Anim Conserv 2012;15(5):480–8.

83. Finke MD. Complete nutrient composition of commercially raised invertebrates used as food for insectivores. Zoo Biol 2002;21:269–85.

84. Finke MD. Complete nutrient content of four species of feeder insects. Zoo Biol 2013;32(1):27–36.

85. Ahmed AA, Sekar S, Oh PY, et al. Hematology and serum biochemistry of captive Sunda pangolin (Manis javanica) in Wildlife Reserves Singapore. J Vet Med Sci 2021;83(2):309–14.

86. Dierenfeld ES, Alcorn HL, Jacobsen KL. Nutrient composition of whole vertebrate prey (excluding fish) fed in zoos. Beltsville: U.S. Department of Agriculture; 2002.

87. Iske CJ, Morris CL, Kappen KL. Evaluation of raw pork as a commercially manufactured diet option for zoo-managed African wildcats (Felis silvestris lybica). Transl Anim Sci 2017;1:397–405.

88. Mazuri. Mazuri® Exotic Feline Diet – Small. 2022a. Available at https://pims.purinamills.com/BusinessLink/media/Mazuri/ProductSheet/5M54.pdf?ext=.pdf. Accessed May 26, 2023.

89. Mazuri. Mazuri® Exotic Canine Diet. 2022b. Available at https://pims.purinamills.com/BusinessLink/media/Mazuri/ProductSheet/5MN2.pdf?ext=.pdf. Accessed May 26, 2023.

90. Mazuri. Mazuri® Insectivore Diet. 2019. Available at https://pims.purinamills.com/BusinessLink/media/Mazuri/ProductSheet/5M6C.pdf?ext=.pdf. Accessed May 26, 2023.

91. Latney LV, Toddes BD, Wyre NR, et al. Effects of various diets on the calcium and phosphorus composition of mealworms (Tenebrio molitor larvae) and superworms (Zophobas morio larvae). Am J Vet Res 2017;78(2):178–85.

92. LaDouceur EEB, Murphy BG, Garner MM, et al. Osteomalacia with hyperostosis in captive lesser hedgehog tenrecs (Echinops telfairi). Vet Pathol 2020;57(6):885–8.

93. Schwitzer C, Kaumanns W. Foraging patterns of free-ranging and captive primates – implications for captive feeding regimens. Zoo Anim Nutr 2003;2:247–65.

94. Mott R, Pellett S, Hedley J. Prevalence and risk factors for dental disease in captive Central bearded dragons (Pogona vitticeps) in the United Kingdom. J Exotic Pet Med 2021;36:1–7.
95. Kristensen L, Malte CL, Malte H, et al. Obesity prolongs induction times in reptiles. Comp Biochem Physiol A 2022;271:111255.
96. Donoghue S. Nutrition of pet amphibians and reptiles. Sem Avian Exotic Pet Med 1998;7(3):148–53.
97. Otunola GA, Oloyede OB, Oladiji AT, et al. Effects of diet-induced hypercholesterolemia on the lipid profile and some enzyme activities in female Wistar rats. Afr. J Biochem Res 2010;4(6):149–54.
98. Sollom HJ, Baron HR. Clinical presentation and disease prevalence of captive central bearded dragons (Pogona vitticeps) at veterinary clinics in Australia. Aust Vet J 2023. Early Access.
99. Barboza PS, Parker KL, Hume ID. Metabolic constituents: water, minerals and vitamins. In Integrative wildlife nutrition. New York: Springer; 2010. p. 157–206.
100. Mayer J, Donnelly TM. Amphibians: nutritional secondary hyperparathyroidism. In Clinical veterinary advisor: birds and exotic pets. St. Louis: Elsevier Saunders; 2013. p. 62–4.
101. Lombardi G, Ziemann E, Banfi G, et al. Physical activity-dependent regulation of parathyroid hormone and calcium-phosphorous metabolism. Int J Molec Sci 2021;21:5388.
102. Wright K. Two common disorders of captive bearded dragons (Pogona vitticeps): nutritional secondary hyperparathyroidism and constipation. J Exotic Pet Med 2008;17(4):267–72.

An Update on Companion Inland Bearded Dragon (*Pogona vitticeps*) Nutrition

Trinita Barboza, DVM, DVSc*, Marjorie Bercier, DMV, DACZM

KEYWORDS

- Bearded dragon • Omnivore • Calcium • Ultraviolet B light • Insect • Vegetation
- Diet • Nutrition

KEY POINTS

- Evidence-based guidelines are lacking on the type, quantity, and frequency of food and supplements offered to captive inland bearded dragons (*Pogona vitticeps*). They are suggested to be opportunistic predators that consume vegetation when arthropods are limited.
- Obesity in captive bearded dragons likely stems from excessive food consumption, high-fat food items such as larval insects, lack of brumation, and a sedentary lifestyle.
- Pet bearded dragons require regular access to fresh and clean water even though they are desert dwellers.
- Ultraviolet B light or natural sunlight is recommended for endogenous vitamin D3 production.
- Most commercial insects and some offered plants have an inverse calcium to phosphorus ratio and are deficient in several vitamins and minerals. Food items should be dusted with pure calcium powder at every feeding and a multivitamin formulated for reptiles including vitamin E, D, and preformed vitamin A on a weekly basis (monthly at minimum). Insects should be gut loaded with an 8% calcium diet for 24 to 48 hours to improve their calcium to phosphorus ratio.

INTRODUCTION

Bearded dragons (*Pogona vitticeps*) are popular pets and are becoming popular research subjects.[1] Understanding their husbandry is vital for their longevity and health in captivity. However, little is known about their specific nutritional requirements making it difficult to establish a balanced diet. Some authors recommend a varied diet of plants and insects to allow the animal to select items that contain required nutrients.[2]

Department of Clinical Sciences, Zoological Companion Animal Medicine Service, Cummings School of Veterinary Medicine at Tufts University, 200 Westboro Road, North Grafton, MA, USA
* Corresponding author.
E-mail address: trinita.barboza@tufts.edu

Vet Clin Exot Anim 27 (2024) 71–84
https://doi.org/10.1016/j.cvex.2023.08.002
1094-9194/24/© 2023 Elsevier Inc. All rights reserved.

The information necessary to make diet recommendations for this species requires analysis of the energy, protein, mineral, and vitamin components that support their maintenance, growth, and reproduction. In addition, evaluation of the composition of the complete diet being consumed by captive bearded dragons, including plant items, invertebrates, pellet formulations, and supplements is required. This information is currently not available as most published data pertain to individual diet components. The complete nutrient composition of various commercially raised invertebrates, as well as methods to manipulate their nutritional value, has been published elsewhere.[3–5] This article reviews the current body of literature on energy and nutritional components consumed by bearded dragons.

DISCUSSION
Energy Balance

The energy balance of a bearded dragon is dependent on multiple factors including caloric intake, metabolism, physical activity, and thermal gradient. Bearded dragons are considered to be omnivorous, opportunistic predators who preferentially select arthropods but consume plant material when insects are limited.[6,7] Older literature suggests that, as larger lizards (>300g), bearded dragons tend toward herbivory as the energetic cost for a large body mass to capture a small insect may significantly reduce the energy profit.[8,9] It was therefore concluded that these animals tend to consume plant material from their habitats with little energy expenditure and opportunistically catch insects.[8,10] Current diet recommendations for captive bearded dragons, based on these studies, suggest that a variety of leafy greens, limited vegetables, and insects would be appropriate.[1,7,11] However, there are no clear guidelines on the target caloric content or composition, and the recommendations on frequency of feeding are variable.[1,7,11] One study evaluated the energy dynamics of celery consumed by bearded dragons and found that the majority of the gained energy went toward metabolic processes and fecal production resulting in a 24% net energy profit.[12] The investigators noted that this energy gain was higher than expected as many considered celery to be a negative calorie food item.[12] Further investigations are required to understand the energy profit of other food items. It is challenging to create recommendations for captive bearded dragons based on free-range animals as their energetics differ due to environmental factors (husbandry) and the composition of vegetation and insects offered.[7,13,14]

In captivity, rapid growth and obesity are noted and is suspected to be secondary to excessive energy intake and reduced energy expenditure.[6,15,16] In clinical practice, most veterinarians body condition score bearded dragons by the muscling around the tail, pelvis, and limbs as well as the size of their coelomic fat pads. Bearded dragons with large tail bases, thick muscling of the limbs, and fat pads that take up a large portion of the coelomic cavity are considered obese. The development of an objective body condition score system is currently being investigated. Some speculate that excessive food consumption, high-fat food items such as larval insects, lack of brumation, and a sedentary lifestyle lead to an energy imbalance resulting in obesity, and possibly hepatic lipidosis.[10,13,16–18] A survey of bearded dragon owners in the United States and Canada highlighted that half the respondents were feeding greater than 50% insects and less than 50% plant material.[18] Though clear nutritional guidelines for captive bearded dragons are lacking, these results suggest that many owners are feeding energy-dense diets to their pets, and it is known than omnivores preferentially select animal material when given a choice.[2] Some veterinarians recommend weighing bearded dragons at home and increasing fiber while reducing animal matter if the pet is obese.[7,16]

The metabolic rate of reptiles is known to be lower than mammals. In a comparison of bearded dragon and rat mitochondria, bearded dragons demonstrated a lower proton permeability of the inner mitochondrial phospholipid membrane due to differences in fatty acid composition resulting in a reduced metabolic rate.[19] It is suspected that this lower metabolic rate indicates a lower energy requirement in bearded dragons. However, a significant variation in rates occurs with reproductive status, season, thermal gradient, and body mass.[16]

In addition to caloric intake and metabolic rate, the thermal gradient plays a vital role in energy balance of ectotherms. Bearded dragons partake in behavioral thermoregulation which has a metabolic cost of locomotion. Depending on the fed or fasted state of the animal, the body temperature, upper and lower set point in the optimal temperature zone, and oxygen consumption are different.[20] During a fasted state, bearded dragons choose a body temperature that is lower by a few degrees within the thermal gradient, have a lower and more narrow optimal thermal range, and consume less oxygen.[20] It is suggested that this voluntary reduction of temperature and oxygen consumption allows for a lower metabolic rate and energy conservation during times of food scarcity, low temperatures, or increased thermoregulatory cost.[20] In a fed state, bearded dragons are thermophilic and choose a higher body temperature within the thermal gradient.[20] The energy cost of moving to a higher temperature and increased oxygen consumption allows for faster digestion, absorption, and assimilation of nutrients to allow for growth, reproduction, and maintenance of physiologic functions.[20–23] The composition of the diet may also play a role in temperature selection as demonstrated in agamid lizards (Amphibolurus nuchalis) who selected higher temperatures to maintain phospholipid membrane fluidity when fed diets high in saturated fatty acids.[24]

Brumation also plays an important role in energy balance, though not common in companion bearded dragons. This metabolic depression is known to occur in free-ranging bearded dragons to survive periods of starvation and cold. Molecular evaluation of these animals has revealed that glucose is their main energy source during brumation, which is dissimilar from mammals who only use lipids.[25–27] This was evidenced by the fact that proteins and genes for glycolysis and glyconeogenesis were upregulated while many lipid and ketone genes involved in fatty acid oxidation were downregulated.[25,26]

Water Balance

For any given living body, water intake and water loss must be balanced to avoid dehydration or overhydration. Terrestrial vertebrates are hyperosmolar to their environment and must constantly fight excessive water loss and subsequent dehydration. The same is true for desert-dwelling species such as bearded dragons, despite the erroneous belief that animals living in arid environments require little to no access to water. In the survey about feeding practices of client-owned bearded dragons, a large portion of respondents did not have water available for their pets.[18] However, authors acknowledged that the survey did not ask if the bearded dragons were being soaked in a shallow dish of water, which may be a preferred method to stimulate drinking in this species.[10]

Water is primarily absorbed through the gastrointestinal tract after eating and drinking, while other sources of water such as cellular metabolism are less clinically relevant.[28] Absorption of environmental water through the cloaca, called "cloacal drinking," has not been clearly evidenced in reptiles and likely represents a misreporting of the literature on this subject.[29,30] Water loss primarily occurs through the kidneys, and can, to a lesser degree, also be lost via the skin (evaporation, sweating), the lungs (breathing), and the gastrointestinal tract (vomiting, diarrhea).[28]

In mammals, water balance and plasma tonicity are tightly regulated by the kidneys which are able to reabsorb water from the glomerular filtrate and produce concentrated urine. Contrary to the mammalian kidney, the reptilian kidney is unable to produce hyperosmotic urine due to the absence of the loop of Henle and the juxtaglomerular apparatus.[31] Most reptiles have evolved with other physiologic mechanisms to maintain plasmatic osmolarity and hydration status as only 30% to 50% of water is absorbed in the proximal tubules, while the rest is absorbed in the distal tubules, colon, cloaca, and in some species, the urinary bladder (not present in bearded dragons).[32] As a terrestrial species, it is reasonable to assume that the preferred nitrogenous waste of P vitticeps is uric acid.

Bearded dragons respond to a state of dehydration by an increase in drinking. A recent study evaluated the diuretic effects of furosemide at 5 and 10 mg/kg subcutaneously every 12 hours for 48 hours in bearded dragons deprived of food and water.[33] Despite not having a loop of Henle, repeated administration of furosemide resulted in diuresis and dehydration, evidenced by weight loss and an increase in packed cell volume, total solids and total proteins (but not uric acid concentration).[33] Twelve hours after the last injection of furosemide, the study subjects were soaked for 5 minutes in warm tap water. Active drinking was observed in almost all bearded dragons that received furosemide which resulted in a significant increase in body weight in comparison to the control group.[33] Weight gain was significantly greater for the 10 mg/kg treatment group compared with the 5 mg/kg treatment group.[33]

Water balance and electrolyte balance are closely related. Interestingly, the plasma osmolarity did not change significantly after inducing a state of dehydration with repetitive administration of furosemide in bearded dragons.[33] The mean measured plasma osmolality of bearded dragons in 1 study was 295.4 ± 9.35 mOsm/kg and 314 ± 9.1 mOsm/kg in another.[33,34] The calculated plasma osmolality via the traditional equation was in poor agreement with the measured plasma osmolality, and so a modified equation $[1.85(Na^+ + K^+)]$ is recommended for this species.[34]

It is generally thought that the scales of lepidosaur reptiles are protective against cutaneous evaporative water loss. A recent study has evaluated evaporative water loss in 3 P vitticeps phenotypes: "wild-types" with normal scalation, "leatherbacks" with scales of reduced prominence, and "silkbacks" or scaleless bearded dragons. Under experimental conditions, silkbacks on average lost water at a slightly higher rate than leatherbacks and at a rate nearly double that of wild-types.[35] This research also highlighted that there was no significant difference in thermal preference between phenotypes.[35] This suggests a lack of plasticity in thermal preference in response to an increase in the rate of evaporative water loss, a strategy where bearded dragons would prioritize immediate thermal benefits over the threat of future dehydration.[35] The reptile veterinarian should take scale phenotype into consideration when making at home recommendations about water access for this species.

Bearded dragons should be provided with access to water at all times, along their thermal gradient. In the face of mild dehydration, soaking is an adequate rehydration method in bearded dragons with appropriate mentation.

Protein/Amino Acids

The amino acid requirements, digestibility, and availability for bearded dragons are unknown. Therefore, species-specific recommendations on the amino acid profile and protein composition of their diet are impossible. For these reasons, the best approximation of the captive diet of bearded dragons is based on the diet composition of their wild counterparts which varies greatly with season, life stage, and prey/plant availability.

The diet of free-ranging bearded dragons, based on stomach content evaluation from 13 adults and 1 subadult specimen, consisted mainly of plant (54.4% of the stomach volume), animal (41.5%), and indigestible (4.1%) materials.[15] However, on a dry matter (DM) basis, animal materials accounted for most of the stomach content weight (61.0%), while plants materials accounted for a lesser proportion (15.7%). The majority of the identified animal materials were invertebrates from the order Isoptera (94.6%), consisting mainly of termites (genus *Drepanotermes*). Crude protein (CP) content from 4 pooled stomach samples was between 41% to 50% of the DM.[15] Knowing that insects generally have a CP content of approximately 60% DM, the CP content of the stomach contents was consistent with a largely insectivorous diet supplemented with plant materials.[15]

Another study evaluating the stomach content of free-ranging bearded dragons found that the plant and animal material content varied with the animal's life stage.[9] The stomach content of adult (n = 6) bearded dragons was predominantly plant materials (93.8% DM), with only 6.2% DM in animal material.[9] In contrast, the stomach contents of juvenile (n = 3) bearded dragons had a lower proportion of plant material (47.6% DM) and a higher proportion of animal material (52.4% DM).[9] That being said, the average body weight of the 3 juvenile bearded dragons included in this study was 3 g, while that of adult bearded dragons was 236.4 g. This study did not evaluate the CP content of the stomach content sampled from these bearded dragons.

Some authors have suggested that a high-protein diet can lead to the formation of a protein-based sludge in the gallbladder of bearded dragons, potentially predisposing them to cholelith formation.[5] This statement is based on the assumption that adult bearded dragons should be fed a predominantly plant-based diet which is lower in CP.[5,9] In a case series of 9 bearded dragons with choleliths, 6 were fed a diet with greater than 80% invertebrates. Further research is needed to evaluate if dietary protein intake is a true predisposing factor for cholelithiasis in this species. Since the diet composition of free-ranging bearded dragons is conflicting, the exact protein and amino acids requirements of bearded dragons remain unknown.[9,15]

Fat/Fatty Acids

The specific fatty acid requirements for bearded dragons have not been described. However, general information for omnivorous reptiles is available. Reptiles are described to store their excess energy as triglycerides (triacylglycerols) regardless of the original macronutrient.[36] Following food consumption, fat, carbohydrates (CHs), and proteins are digested and absorbed. The dietary triglycerides are transported by enteromicrons to peripheral tissues for storage or oxidation.[36] Excess amino acids and CHs are transported to the liver where they undergo lipogenesis to synthetize triglycerides for export and storage.[36] These triglycerides are later metabolized to meet energy demands.[36] Excess glucose can also be converted into glycogen for storage in the liver as well.[36]

Several publications exist on the crude fat content and fatty acid composition of insects. They generally suggest that larval insects are higher in fat, particularly saturated fatty acids (eg, palmitic acid or lauric acid), while adult insects are lower in fat and contain more polyunsaturated fatty acids.[3,4,17,37,38] For insects that do not pupate, such as the house cricket, the fat content increases throughout the nymphal stage and then slowly declines in adulthood.[39] Many factors, in addition to life stage, play a role in the fat content and fatty acid composition of each insect including the species, sex, diet, temperature, and photoperiod.[40,41] For example, the house cricket is one of the few species of insects that are able to synthesize linoleic and linolenic acids (polyunsaturated fatty acids); they have increased saturated fatty acids at higher environmental temperatures, and females have a higher fat content compared to males.[4,41,42] These variations in fatty acid composition likely make it challenging to recommend specific insects for consumption.

Differences have also been highlighted between commercially raised insects and wild insects. Commercial crickets have a higher fat content and lower levels of omega-3 fatty acids and linolenic acid which is suggested to be secondary to their grain-based diets and reduced activity compared to wild crickets.[3,4,37,43,44] Additionally, there are several differences in vitamin and mineral components between commercial and wild insects discussed in the following paragraphs.

The specific fat content of various larval and adult insects has been described with superworms (*Zophobas morio*) having some of the highest percent fat on a DM basis (22.1%) and silkworms (*Bombyx mori*) having the lowest fat on a DM basis (1.4%).[3,14,37,43,45–47] Studies in western fence lizards (*Sceloporus occidentalis*) and leopard geckos (*Eublepharis macularius*) demonstrated that when these lizards were fed equal weights of mealworms or crickets, they had increased feed conversion efficiency and weight gain with mealworms since they contained more fat.[48,49] From these studies, it is apparent that commercial insects, particularly larval insects, are higher in energy. These insects could be a risk factor for obesity and hepatic lipidosis in bearded dragons when offered in abundance year-round, as is common practice in captivity.[18] Though lower fat insects are recommended by authors for obese animals, a variety of larval and adult insects are recommended for balance in other nutritional factors such as minerals and amino acids.[4] Active (adult) insects also improve foraging behavior and encourage activity in captive bearded dragons who likely have an abundance of caloric intake and reduced activity.[50] Lastly, overconsumption of CHs from plant material should also be considered as a risk factor for obesity due to de novo lipogenesis.

Carbohydrates: Sugars, Starches, Fibers

The CH requirements of *P vitticeps*, as well as the CH content of their natural diet, are unknown. Since CH content appears to be minimal in insects, it is generally accepted that most of the CH consumed by omnivorous reptiles comes from plant material.[3,4] Neither of the previous ecological studies (see Protein/Amino Acids) investigated the CH content of the retrieved bearded dragons' stomach contents.[9,15] The composition of vegetation in the wild is different from commercially available vegetables, which are low in minerals and fiber and high in simple CHs.[9,13,18,51] The differences between wild and commercial vegetation raise questions about whether store-bought produce accurately represents plant matter eaten in the wild.[18]

In the survey on feeding practices of bearded dragon owners, fruits were offered by 70.5% of owners but were offered in small portions (<25%) by the majority.[18] The presence of fruit in the diet is significantly associated with the presence of dental abnormalities and disease in captive bearded dragons.[52] The odds of having dental abnormalities and disease are higher (odds ratio 2.68; 1.61–4.46) for bearded dragons with fruit present in the diet.[52] There was no significant association between the presence of dental abnormalities and disease and the amount of vegetable matter in the diet, nor with the presence of individual insects.[52] This suggests that the high sugar content and acidity of fruit may play an important role in the etiology of dental disease in bearded dragons.[52]

While no evidence-based recommendations on dietary CH content can be made, plant matter in the form of commercially available vegetable can be offered to captive bearded dragons without obvious adverse health effects. Fruits should be avoided and leafy greens should be favored.

Vitamins

Vitamin D

The requirement for vitamin D3 in the prevention of metabolic bone disease is well-known. In a study evaluating a variety of lizards including *P barbata* with natural sun exposure, calcidiol was found to be the most indicative of vitamin D status, and plasma concentration were reported to be 105 ± 12 nmol/L.[53] Bearded dragons are able to synthetize endogenous vitamin D3 through ultraviolet B (UVB) exposure (290–320 nm) which can remain stable for 83 days after discontinuation of UVB.[54]

In the survey on feeding practices of bearded dragon, the majority of owners provided UVB exposure in addition to oral vitamin D supplementation in their calcium powder.[18] Though the findings were consistent with some recommendations in the literature, frequent supplementation of unknown quantity of oral vitamin D could risk toxicity and unregulated calcium absorption resulting in dystrophic mineralization, so pure calcium supplementation is recommended.[51,55,56]

Studies have compared the efficacy of oral vitamin D3 supplementation to UVB bulb exposure, and the results are conflicting.[6,57] One study indicated oral vitamin D3 supplementation was ineffective compared to a UVB bulb while the other study found both to be adequate to maintain calcidiol levels.[6,57] These conflicting results could have been due to differences in bulbs used as studies have indicated that not all UVB bulbs are equivalent.[58,59] These studies evaluating various UVB bulbs have indicated that natural sun exposure is superior to artificial UVB exposure and that the spectral power of distribution of the bulbs plays a key role in their efficacy.[58,59] Two Zoo Med bulbs, a Reptisun 5.0 UVB bulb with 2 hours of exposure, and a full spectrum light-emitting diode (LED) 7W UVB bulb with 12-hour exposure, are reported to be effective, though the LED bulb is superior due to the spectrum of the bulb.[6,59] In addition to bulb efficacy, phenotypic variations must be considered as scaleless bearded dragons choose lower levels of UVB.[35]

Vitamin D concentrations in insects has also been evaluated. Wild-caught insects are found to have a large variability in vitamin D concentrations, though higher than commercially raised insects.[37] When commercially raised house crickets and yellow mealworms are exposed to UVB, they are able to synthesize vitamin D3 and therefore increase their concentrations.[60] However, it is not common practice to provide feeder insects UVB in pet stores or in homes, and UVB or sun exposure to bearded dragons is thought to be sufficient for their vitamin D levels.

Vitamin A

Vitamin A requirements in bearded dragons are also unknown at this time. As omnivores, they can consume both the biologically active form of vitamin A (retinoids) through animal material as well as the provitamin (carotenoids) through plants.[61] Based on green iguanas (*Iguana iguana*), it is suggested that the most effective carotenoids in reptiles are lutein and canthaxanthin.[62] Though herbivores can synthesize carotenoids into retinoids, many carnivores and omnivores are suggested to lack the enzyme required.[61,63] While it is unknown if a bearded dragon can synthesize retinoids from carotenoids, evidence exists that the insectivorous panther chameleon (*Furcifer pardalis*) is able to do so effectively.[64]

Evaluation of carotenoids in plants and insects have indicated higher levels of carotenoids are present in dark green and yellow plants and higher levels of carotenoids are present in wild insects due to their diet.[4,44,65] Insects only synthesize retinoids in their compound eye resulting in overall low levels and absent levels for those that lack compound eyes.[66] Since the bearded dragon's ability to synthesize retinoids form carotenoids is unknown, authors suggest gut loading insects with an active form of vitamin A.

Vitamin E

The mean plasmatic concentration (23.23 ± 18.63 pmol/L) of vitamin E (α-tocopherol) has been reported in clinically healthy bearded dragons.[67] These concentrations did not significantly differ between various diets that were supplemented with a multivitamin.[67] However, no study outlines the minimum nutritional requirement for a bearded dragon or the clinical signs or metabolic derangements associated with its deficiencies. Sources of vitamin E for bearded dragons include insects and some plant material.

The nutritional composition of insects has highlighted that vitamin E concentrations tend to be variable in insects depending on their diet, though higher in wild insects.[4,68] High dietary supplementation of vitamin E to insects resulted in higher levels of vitamin E incorporated into the tissues.[37]

Minerals

Though no specific guidelines have been created for bearded dragons, calcium supplementation has been studied extensively in insect-eating lizards. Insufficient dietary calcium is a leading cause of metabolic bone disease in reptiles. A retrospective study of bearded dragons indicated that almost 58% of animals had an abnormal calcium-to-phosphorus (Ca/P) ratio with the majority having hypocalcemia and a few having hyperphosphatemia.[69] Though not reported in bearded dragons, oversupplementation of calcium in chelonians has resulted in poor growth, deficiencies of zinc, copper, and iodine, and dystrophic mineralization in extreme cases.[7,70,71]

Though complete pelleted diets exist, they are cautiously recommended as they may not be readily accepted and the nutritional requirements for captive bearded dragons are debated as a standard for nutritional adequacy has not been established.[7,10] A study evaluating 15 commercial diets found all of them to have excessive iron and some of them to have excessive calcium.[72]

Common food items of bearded dragons including commercially raised insects and some plants have an inverse Ca/P ratio (0.08–0.30:1).[14,44,73] In the recent years, phoenix worms or black soldier fly larvae (*Hermetia illucens)* have been popularized as insects with adequate calcium content due to their mineralized exoskeleton.[4] These insects are noted to have a 2.6:1 Ca/P ratio when fasted and are also rich in magnesium, potassium, iron, manganese, and zinc.[73] Since the majority of the calcium is bound in the exoskeleton, the bioavailability of this calcium has been investigated.[73–75] These studies indicated that reptiles that chew the insects had a higher bioavailability of the calcium though the digestibility still remained low (43%).[74,75]

Other important minerals include phosphorus, sodium, potassium, and trace minerals such as zinc, copper, magnesium, and selenium. The phosphorus of insects is believed to be bioavailable, while much of the phosphorus in plants is nondigestible phytates.[4,76] Sodium, potassium, and other trace mineral concentrations in insects are speculated to meet nutritional requirements for most animals.[3,4,43,44]

Due to the well-known vitamin and mineral deficiencies in commercially raised insects, dusting and gut loading are recommended. A study evaluating the efficacy of dusting crickets with calcium and multivitamins prior to feeding found that more than 50% of the dust is removed by the crickets within 2.5 minutes.[77] However, dusting is still advised though the recommendations are unclear and range from daily to once a week for pure calcium and weekly to monthly for multivitamins.[7,10,40,51] Since calcium salts inhibit phosphorus absorption, dusting likely should occur every time food is offered to improve the Ca/P ratio.[10] Dusting of plant material is also recommended due to the inverse Ca/P ratio of some plants though recommendations on quantity is lacking. Authors recommend daily dusting of food items with pure calcium and weekly dusting with a multivitamin.

In addition to dusting, gut loading is considered key in improving the concentrations of limited nutrients in the insect gut which accounts for 4% to 7% of its body weight.[43,78] Various studies have proven the efficacy of gut loading by demonstrating a variation of calcium, iron, zinc and manganese content in black soldier fly prepupae fed different diets and increasing zinc concentrations in housefly pupae that were fed diets supplemented with zinc chloride.[79,80] The current consensus for gut-loading insects is to provide insects with a diet consisting of 8% calcium for 24 to 48 hours to improve the Ca/P ratio.[81] These high-calcium diets should only be fed short-term as they are unpalatable to crickets and can lead to high mortality due to the nutritional imbalance.[7] Various gut-loading diets are marketed with only a few proven to be efficacious including Fluker's High-Calcium Mealworm Diet for mealworms, T-Rex Calcium Plus for crickets, and Mazuri High Calcium Cricket Diet for crickets, mealworms, and superworms.[73,82–84] Though most gut-loading studies primarily focus on improving the Ca/P ratio, other vitamins and minerals are present in these formulas to account for known imbalances.

SUMMARY

Though there is a significant amount of literature on various aspects of bearded dragon energy balance and nutrition, a consensus on the minimal requirements or target caloric intake is currently lacking. Until evidence-based recommendations are available, the authors recommend that bearded dragons be offered diets high in fiber (leafy greens) with a variety of insects and a limited amount of simple CHs and fatty larval insects. These diets should be dusted with pure calcium powder when offered and a multivitamin on occasion. Commercial insects should be gut loaded with a proven diet to improve their known vitamin and mineral deficiencies. Until clear recommendations can be made for oral vitamin D supplementation, UVB bulbs or natural sunlight is preferred. In addition, water should always be available in a large vessel so that the bearded dragon can soak and drink. Further investigations are required for exercise and brumation recommendations.

CLINICS CARE POINTS

- Proven gut-loading diets for insects include Fluker's High Calcium Mealworm Diet, T-Rex Calcium Plus, and Mazuri High Calcium Cricket Diet.

- Fruits are a significant risk factor for dental disease in bearded dragons.

- More than half of captive bearded dragons presenting to clinics in Europe had abnormal Ca/P ratios.

- Natural sun exposure is superior to UVB bulb exposure for vitamin D3 synthesis.

- Larval insects tend to be higher in fat, with superworms, a popular food item for bearded dragons, having some of the highest fat percentages on a DM basis.

- The mineralized exoskeleton of phoenix worms has increased bioavailability in reptiles that chew the insect.

- Provide at least 50% high-fiber plant matter dusted in pure calcium and less than 50% adult and lower fat larval insects gut loaded for 24 to 48 hours with an 8% calcium diet and dusted with pure calcium. Provide multivitamins on a weekly basis, or monthly at minimum. Provide a water dish large enough to soak and drink.

DISCLOSURE

Authors do not have any commercial or financial conflicts of interest or funding sources for this article.

REFERENCES

1. Cannon M. Husbandry and veterinary aspects of the bearded dragon (Pogona spp.) in Australia. Semin Avian Exot Pet Med 2003;12:205–14.
2. Oonincx D, van Leeuwen J. Evidence-based reptile housing and nutrition. Vet Clin North Am Exot Anim Pract 2017;20:885–98.
3. Finke MD. Complete nutrient composition of commercially raised invertebrates used as food for insectivores. Zoo Biol 2002;21:269–85.
4. Oonincx DGAB, Finke MD. Nutritional value of insects and ways to manipulate their composition. J Insects Food Feed 2021;7:639–59.
5. Gimmel A, Kempf H, Öfner S, et al. Cholelithiasis in adult bearded dragons: retrospective study of nine adult bearded dragons (Pogona vitticeps) with cholelithiasis between 2013 and 2015 in southern Germany. J Anim Physiol Anim Nutr 2017;101:122–6.
6. Oonincx DGAB, Stevens Y, van den Borne JJGC, et al. Effects of vitamin D3 supplementation and UVb exposure on the growth and plasma concentration of vitamin D3 metabolites in juvenile bearded dragons (Pogona vitticeps). Comp Biochem Physiol B Biochem Mol Biol 2010;156:122–8.
7. Donoghue S, McKeown S. Nutrition of captive reptiles. Vet Clin North Am Exot Anim Pract 1999;2:69–91.
8. Pough F. Lizard energetics and diet. Ecology 1973;54:837–44.
9. MacMillen RE, Augee ML, Ellis BA. Thermal ecology and diet of some xerophilous lizards from western New South Wales. J Arid Environ 1989;16:193–201.
10. Boyer TH, Scott PW. Nutrition. In: Divers SJ, Stahl SJ, editors. Mader's reptile and amphibian medicine and surgery. 3rd edition. St. Louis: Elsevier; 2019. p. 201–23.
11. de Vosjoli PM. A simple system for raising juvenile bearded dragons indoors. Vivarium 1996;7:42–55.
12. Buddemeyer K, Alexander A. and Secor S. Negative calorie foods: An empirical examination of what is fact or fiction, bioRxiv, 2019, 586958. Avaliable at: https://doi.org/10.1101/586958. Accessed May 23, 2023.
13. Boyer TH, Scott PW. Nutritional diseases. In: Divers SJ, Stahl SJ, editors. Mader's reptile and amphibian medicine and surgery. 3rd edition. St. Louis: Elsevier; 2019. p. 932–50.
14. Finke MD. Complete nutrient content of four species of commercially available feeder insects fed enhanced diets during growth. Zoo Biol 2015;34:554–64.
15. Oonincx DG, van Leeuwen JP, Hendriks WH, et al. The diet of free-roaming Australian Central bearded dragons (Pogona vitticeps). Zoo Biol 2015;34:271–7.
16. Mans C, Braun J. Update on common nutritional disorders of captive reptiles. Vet Clin North Am Exot Anim Pract 2014;17:369–95.
17. Barker D, Fitzpatrick MP, Dierenfeld ES. Nutrient composition of selected whole invertebrates. Zoo Biol 1998;17:123–34.
18. Barboza TK, Abood SK, Beaufrère H. Survey of feeding practices and supplement use in pet inland bearded dragons (Pogona vitticeps) of the United States and Canada. J Herpetol Med Surg 2022;32:187–97.
19. Brand MD, Couture P, Else PL, et al. Evolution of energy metabolism. Proton permeability of the inner membrane of liver mitochondria is greater in a mammal than in a reptile. Biochem J 1991;275:81–6.

20. Plummer, AC. Thermal preference and the effects of food availability on components of fitness in the bearded dragon, Pogona vitticeps. In: University of Ottawa Theses, 1910-2010. 2009. Avaliable at: https://doi.org/10.20381/ruor-12499. Accessed May 1, 2023.
21. Angilletta MJ. Thermal and physiological constraints on energy assimilation in a widespread lizard (Sceloporus undulatus). Ecology 2001;82:3044–56.
22. Wang T, Zaar M, Arvedsen S, et al. Effects of temperature on the metabolic response to feeding in Python molurus. Comp Biochem Physiol Mol Integr Physiol 2002;133:519–27.
23. Kleiber M. The fire of life. An introduction to animal energetics. New York: Wiley; 1961.
24. Geiser F, Learmonth R. Dietary fats, selected body temperature and tissue fatty acid composition of agamid lizzards. J Comp Physiol B 1994;164:55–61.
25. Capraro A, O'Meally D, Waters SA, et al. Waking the sleeping dragon: gene expression profiling reveals adaptive strategies of the hibernating reptile Pogona vitticeps. BMC Genom 2019;20:460.
26. Capraro A, O'Meally D, Waters SA, et al. MicroRNA dynamics during hibernation of the Australian central bearded dragon (Pogona vitticeps). Sci Rep 2020;10: 17854.
27. Dark J. Annual lipid cycles in hibernators: integration of physiology and behavior. Annu Rev Nutr 2005;25:469–97.
28. JL L. Dehydration. In: Merck Manual Consumer Version. 2022. Available at: https://www.merckmanuals.com/home/hormonal-and-metabolic-disorders/water-balance/dehydration. Accessed May 23, 2023.
29. Gibbons PM. Critical care nutrition and fluid therapy in reptiles. In: Proceeding of the 15th Annual International Veteirnary Emergency & Critical Care Symposium. 2009. Avaliable at: https://www.avianexoticvetcare.com/userfiles/Reptile_Critical_Care_IVECCS_2009.pdf.
30. Minnich J. The use of water. In: Gans C, Pough F, editors. Biology of the Reptilia. London and New York: Academic Press; 1982. p. 325–95.
31. Ford SS, Bradshaw SD. Kidney function and the role of arginine vasotocin in three agamid lizards from habitats of differing aridity in Western Australia. Gen Comp Endocrinol 2006;147:62–9.
32. Holz PH. Anatomy and physiology of the reptile renal system. Vet Clin North Am Exot Anim Pract 2020;23:103–14.
33. Parkinson LA, Mans C. Effects of furosemide administration to water-deprived inland bearded dragons (Pogona vitticeps). Am J Vet Res 2018;79:1204–8.
34. Dallwig RK, Mitchell MA, Acierno MJ. Determination of plasma osmolality and agreement between measured and calculated values in healthy adult bearded dragons (Pogona vitticeps). J Herpetol Med Surg 2010;20:69–73.
35. Sakich NB, Tattersall GJ. Bearded dragons (Pogona vitticeps) with reduced scalation lose water faster but do not have substantially different thermal preferences. J Exp Biol 2021;224:jeb234427.
36. Price ER. The physiology of lipid storage and use in reptiles. Biol Rev Camb Philos Soc 2017;92:1406–26.
37. Finke M. Complete nutrient content of three species of wild caught insects, pallid-winged grasshopper, rhinoceros beetles and white-lined sphinx moth. J Insects Food Feed 2015;1:1–12.
38. Ewald N, Vidakovic A, Langeland M, et al. Fatty acid composition of black soldier fly larvae (Hermetia illucens) – Possibilities and limitations for modification through diet. Waste Manag 2020;102:40–7.

39. Lipsitz EY, McFarlane JE. Analysis of lipid during the life cycle of the house cricket, Acheta domesticus. Insect Biochem 1971;1:446–60.

40. Finke MD, Oonincx DGAB. Nutrient content of insects. In: van Huis A, Tomberlin JK, editors. Insects as food and feed: from production to consumption. Wageningen: Wageningen Academic Press; 2017. p. 290–316.

41. Kulma M, Kouřimská L, Plachý V, et al. Effect of sex on the nutritional value of house cricket, Acheta domestica L. Food Chem 2019;272:267–72.

42. Borgeson CE, Blomquist GJ. Subcellular location of the Δ12 desaturase rules out bacteriocyte contribution to linoleate biosynthesis in the house cricket and the American cockroach. Insect Biochem Mol Biol 1993;23:297–302.

43. Finke MD. Complete nutrient content of four species of feeder insects. Zoo Biol 2013;32:27–36.

44. Oonincx DG, Dierenfeld ES. An investigation into the chemical composition of alternative invertebrate prey. Zoo Biol 2012;31:40–54.

45. Landry SV, Defoliart GR, Sunde ML. Larval protein quality of six species of Lepidoptera (Saturniidae, Sphingidae, Noctuidae). J Econ Entomol 1986;79:600–4.

46. Yang LF, Siriamornpun S, Li D. Polyunsaturated fatty acid content of edible insects in thailand. J Food Lipids 2006;13:277–85.

47. Donoghue S, Langenberg J. Nutrition. In: Mader DR, editor. Reptile medicine and surgery. 1st edition. Philadelphia: WB Saunders; 1996. p. 148–74.

48. Rich CN, Talent LG. The effects of prey species on food conversion efficiency and growth of an insectivorous lizard. Zoo Biol 2008;27:181–7.

49. Gauthier C, Lesbarrères D. Growth rate variation in captive species: the case of Leopard Geckos, Eublepharis macularius. Herpetol Conserv Biol 2010;5:449–55.

50. Januszczak IS, Bryant Z, Tapley B, et al. Is behavioural enrichment always a success? Comparing food presentation strategies in an insectivorous lizard (Plica plica). Appl Anim Behav Sci 2016;183:95, 03.

51. Raiti P. Husbandry, diseases, and veterinary care of the bearded dragon (Pogona vitticeps). J Herpetol Med Surg 2012;22:117–31.

52. Mott R, Pellett S, Hedley J. Prevalence and risk factors for dental disease in captive central bearded dragons (Pogona vitticeps) in the United Kingdom. J Exot Pet Med 2021;36:1–7.

53. Laing CJ, Fraser DR. The vitamin D system in iguanian lizards. Comp Biochem Physiol B Biochem Mol Biol 1999;123:373–9.

54. Oonincx DGAB, van de Wal MD, Bosch G, et al. Blood vitamin D3 metabolite concentrations of adult female bearded dragons (Pogona vitticeps) remain stable after ceasing UVb exposure. Comp Biochem Physiol B Biochem Mol Biol 2013;165: 196–200.

55. Cannizzo SA, Reppert A, Ward A, et al. Metastatic mineralization in a zoologic collection of spot-tailed earless lizards (holbrookiaspp.). J Zoo Wildl Med 2023; 54:175–84.

56. Vergneau-Grosset C, Carmel ÉN, Raulic J, et al. Vitamin D toxicosis in a blue-tongued skink (Tiliqua scincoides) presented with epistaxis and tongue discoloration. J Herpetol Med Surg 2021;30:224–31.

57. Hetényi N, Sátorhelyi T, Kovács S, et al. Effects of two dietary vitamin and mineral supplements on the growth and health of Hermann's tortoise (Testudo hermanni). Berl Munch Tierarztl Wochenschr 2014;127:251–6.

58. Diehl JJE, Baines FM, Heijboer AC, et al. A comparison of UVb compact lamps in enabling cutaneous vitamin D synthesis in growing bearded dragons. J Anim Physiol Anim Nutr 2018;102:308–16.

59. Cusack L, Rivera S, Lock B, et al. Effects of a light-emitting diode on the production of cholecalciferol and associated blood parameters in the bearded dragon (pogona vitticeps). J Zoo Wildl Med 2017;48:1120–6.

60. Oonincx D, van Keulen P, Finke MD, et al. Evidence of vitamin D synthesis in insects exposed to UVb light. Sci Rep 2018;8:10807.

61. Wedekind KJ, Kats L, Yu S, et al. Microinutrients: Minerals and Vitamins. In: Hand MS, Thatcher CD, Remillard RL, et al, editors. Small animal clinical nutrition. 5th edition. Topeka: Mark Morris Institute; 2010. p. 107–48.

62. Raila J, Schuhmacher A, Gropp J, et al. Selective absorption of carotenoids in the common green iguana (Iguana iguana). Comp Biochem Physiol Mol Integr Physiol 2002;132:513–8.

63. Wilkinson SL. Reptile wellness management. Vet Clin North Am Exot Anim Pract 2015;18:281–304.

64. Dierenfeld ES, Norkus EB, Carroll K, et al. Carotenoids, vitamin A, and vitamin E concentrations during egg development in panther chameleons (Furcifer pardalis). Zoo Biol 2002;21:295–303.

65. Ferguson GW, Jones JRE, Gehrmann WH, et al. Indoor husbandry of the panther chameleon Chamaeleo [Furcifer] pardalis: Effects of dietary vitamins A and D and ultraviolet irradiation on pathology and life-history traits. Zoo Biol 1996;15: 279–99.

66. von Lintig J. Metabolism of carotenoids and retinoids related to vision. J Biol Chem 2012;287:1627–34.

67. Paoloni MC, Freeman LM, Mertz GA, et al. Glutathione peroxidase activity and vitamin E concentrations in bearded dragons, Pogona vitticeps. J Herpetol Med Surg 2000;10:21–5.

68. Pennino M, Dierenfeld ES, Behler JL. Retinol, α-tocopherol and proximate nutrient composition of invertebrates used as feed. Int Zoo Yearb 1991;30:143–9.

69. Schmidt-Ukaj S, Hochleithner M, Richter B, et al. A survey of diseases in captive bearded dragons: A retrospective study of 529 patients. Vet Med (Praha) 2017; 62:508–15.

70. Fledelius B, Jørgensen GW, Jensen HE, et al. Influence of the calcium content of the diet offered to leopard tortoises (Geochelone pardalis). Vet Rec 2005;156: 831–5.

71. Stancel CF, Dierenfeld ES, Schoknecht PA. Calcium and phosphorus supplementation decreases growth, but does not induce pyramiding, in young red-eared sliders, Trachemys scripta elegans. Zoo Biol 1998;17:17–24.

72. Kik M, Dorrestein G, Beynen A. Evaluation of 15 commercial diets and their possible relation to metabolic diseases in different species of reptiles. Verh ber Erkrg Zootiere 2003;41:1–5.

73. Boykin K, Mitchell MA. The value of black soldier fly larvae (Hermetia illucens) as a food source: A review. J Herpetol Med Surg 2021;31:3–11.

74. Boykin KL, Carter RT, Butler-Perez K, et al. Digestibility of black soldier fly larvae (Hermetia illucens) fed to leopard geckos (Eublepharis macularius). PLoS One 2020;15:e0232496.

75. Dierenfeld ES, King J. Digestibility and mineral availability of phoenix worms, Hermetia illucens, ingested by mountain chicken frogs, Leptodactylus fallax. J Herpetol Med Surg 2008;18:100–5.

76. Dashefsky HS, Anderson DL, Tobin EN, et al. Face fly pupae: A potential feed supplement for poultry. Environ Entomol 1976;5:680–2.

77. Li H, Vaughan MJ, Browne RK. A complex enrichment diet improves growth and health in the endangered wyoming toad (Bufo baxteri). Zoo Biol 2009;28: 197–213.
78. Finke M. Gut loading to enhance the nutrient content of insects as food for reptiles: A mathematical approach. Zoo Biol 2003;22:147–62.
79. Spranghers T, Ottoboni M, Klootwijk C, et al. Nutritional composition of black soldier fly (Hermetia illucens) prepupae reared on different organic waste substrates. J Sci Food Agric 2017;97:2594–600.
80. Maryański M, Kramarz P, Laskowski R, et al. Decreased energetic reserves, morphological changes and accumulation of metals in carabid beetles (Poecilus cupreus L.) Exposed to zinc- or cadmium-contaminated food. Ecotoxicology 2002;11:127–39.
81. Allen ME, Oftedal OT. Dietary manipulation of the calcium content of feed crickets. J Zoo Wildl Med 1989;20:26–33.
82. Finke M, Dunham S, Kwabi C. Evaluation of four dry commercial gut loading products for improving the calcium content of crickets, Acheta domesticus. J Herpetol Med Surg 2005;15:7–12.
83. Latney LV, Toddes BD, Wyre NR, et al. Evaluation of nutrient composition of common invertebrate feeders fed different supplemental diets. In: Proceedings of the Eighth Conference on Zoo and Wildlife Nutrition, AZA Nutrition Advisory Group, Tulsa, OK. 2009. Available at: https://nagonline.net/wp-content/uploads/2014/03/04_LatneyInverts.pdf. Accessed May 1, 2023.
84. Brooks M, Harris G. Gut-loading diet evaluation for crickets (Acheta domesticus), mealworms (Tenebrio molitor), and superworms (Zophobas morio) for the purposes of optimizing institutional protocols. In: Proceedings of the Twelfth Conference on Zoo and Wildlife Nutrition, Zoo and Wildlife Nutrition Foundation and AZA Nutrition Advisory Group, Frisco, TX. 2017. Available at: https://nagonline.net/wp-content/uploads/2019/08/Brooks2-Brooks-Harris-2017-Gut-loading-diet-evaluation-for-crickets-mealworms-superworms.pdf. Accessed May 23, 2023.

Important Factors in Chelonian Nutrition

Matthew A. Brooks, MS, PhD[a,b],*

KEYWORDS

- Chelonian • Freshwater turtle • Turtle • Tortoise • Nutrition • Testudines

KEY POINTS

- Feeding Ecology is the primary factor in determing how different species of chelonians are fed.
- Body condition scoring is a difficult, but essential, metric in monitoring the health of chelonians.
- The diet of chelonians in human care should consist of a species appropriate formulated commerical diet along with other natural diet items.

INTRODUCTION

The collective term of Chelonians generally refers to the order of reptiles known as Testudines. This order consists of a myriad of species of shelled animals we know generally as turtles and tortoises. Within this order there are approximately 360 different species that are living today. For the purposes of this article, the focus will be on the nutrition of the animals cared for in a captive setting. The decisions regarding the diet of the animals kept in human care is of the utmost importance for all animals but even more so for those animals that are considered endangered or threatened, such as the western pond turtle, box turtle, alligator snapping turtle, desert tortoise, and gopher tortoise, to name a few. Many institutions are working hard to help with the recovery of these animals through captive populations. Aside from these, there are also several popular species that are kept in the pet trade such as red-eared sliders, painted turtles, musk turtles, leopard tortoises, African spurred tortoises, and red-footed tortoises. These animals deserve the same level of care as the threatened species, and they are going to be the ones that will be most seen by those in the veterinary field due to the sheer volume of animals that are held in the private sector.

Although these turtles and tortoises can be taxonomically divided among several orders, this article will divide them simply, nutritionally, into three main categories:

[a] Animalis Nutrition Consulting, LLC, IN 46077, USA; [b] NomNomNow, Inc, Nashville, TN 37218, USA
* Animalis Nutrition Consulting, LLC, Zionsville, IN 46077.
E-mail address: mbrooks@animalisnutrition.com

Vet Clin Exot Anim 27 (2024) 85–100
https://doi.org/10.1016/j.cvex.2023.07.004
1094-9194/24/© 2023 Elsevier Inc. All rights reserved.

freshwater aquatic turtles, terrestrial turtles, and tortoises. Each of these categories of chelonian inhabit a specific ecological and, thus, nutritional niche, which means the diets and methods for feeding them need to be adapted accordingly. Further, care must be taken to ensure the animals maintain an appropriate body condition, which can be maintained by monitoring intake, growth rate, and physical attributes that are indicators if an animal is under- or over-weight. There is a dearth of peer-reviewed studies regarding chelonian nutrition; however, this article will cover, to the best of its ability, the important factors that should be considered in any veterinary practice when working to provide the best nutrition for its chelonian clients.

Feeding Ecology

Freshwater turtles spend very little time on land. They eat, sleep, and mate in the water, only coming out of their ponds to bask in the sun or to lay eggs. In fact, these animals eat exclusively in the water and will not and cannot eat on dry land. Their food must be fed in the water. The feeding strategy of these turtles can evolve over the lifespan of the animal. When they emerge as hatchlings, turtles, like most animals, start out in a rapid growth phase that requires a diet higher in readily digestible protein and lower in fibrous matter. In this regard, young turtles begin their lives as carnivores. Their diet will start out consisting of insects, annelids, crustaceans, and fish. In the wild, these appropriately sized prey are generally larval insects or immature fish, which are themselves lower in fat and higher in protein. Some species, such as the snapping turtles (*Chelydridae* spp.) and most side-necked turtles (*Pelusios* spp.) will remain primarily carnivorous over their entire lifespan. However, several species in the family Emydidae shift to more omnivory as they mature and their rapid growth phase subsides. Some even switch to a completely herbivorous diet. They will subsist on vegetation that includes algae, leaves, stems, grasses, sedges, and even fruit that falls into the freshwater in which they reside.[1]

Terrestrial turtles are included in the Emydidae family. They are distinctly different from freshwater turtles in that they spend much of their life on land. They can be found in and around water such as ponds and marshes as they prefer a moister environment where they can soak and bury in the moist soils.[2] Like the freshwater turtles, they too start as carnivores and become more omnivorous with age. These animals are very opportunistic feeders that will eat most things that they can forage, scavenge, or catch. Their diet consists of insects, annelids, gastropods, fruits, forbes, other vegetation, and even carrion.

Tortoises inhabit a completely different environment, but, using the same body structures, they have adapted to this world of theirs that is devoid of water. There are, of course, tortoises that do live in very lush environments with an abundance of water, but their design allows them to conserve much of that water by extracting as much it as possible from the food they eat. Most tortoises are 100% herbivorous from the start of their life until the end of it; however, as there are exceptions to every rule, there are tortoises that will consume small worms and larval insects soon after hatching for the extra protein. What vegetation tortoises eat depends entirely on the environment they inhabit. These items range anywhere from cactus pads and flowers, to grasses and hays, to forbes, fruits, and roots. Still, there are some tortoises, such as the Red-footed tortoise, that are omnivorous, and such as the terrestrial turtles, opportunistically feed on different animal proteins as a smaller part of their diet.

Digestive physiology

Chelonians have developed very simple digestive morphology regarding the ingestion and digestion of food. This system is based on the digestive principle that they are in

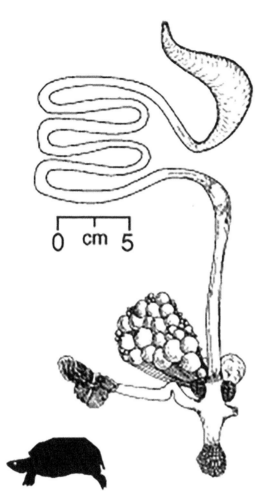

Fig. 1. Blanding's Turtle (*Pseudemys scripta*) digestive tract (Stevens and Hume, 1995).

no hurry to pass food through their digestive tract. In fact, the retention time of larger animals, such as Aldabra tortoises, can be as long as 23 to 49 days.[3] However, this is dependent upon the type of diet and the season. Normal transit time for freshwater turtles has been measured between 3 and 10 days.[4]

Chelonians are the only reptiles to lack teeth. This lack of dentition means they do not have a method to masticate their food. Instead, they make use of a horny beak to bite and cut at their food. Food is swallowed whole or in large pieces to be digested. **Fig. 1** shows the simple gut of a Blanding's turtle, which is an omnivorous aquatic turtle. The stomach is a glandular stomach that secretes digestive acids and enzymes to break down the high protein diet. The small intestine is longer per body size than that of tortoises, and there is not as clear a definition between the small and large intestine, although an ileocolic valve or sphincter does separate the two sections. At the end of the colon the reproductive system connects with the digestive system at the cloaca.[5]

Compared to the more carnivorous/omnivorous diet of turtles to the mostly herbivorous diet of tortoises has manifested into a shorter small intestine but a larger more developed large intestine than their aquatic cousins (**Fig. 2**). This developed large

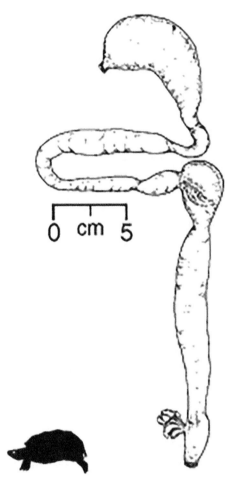

Fig. 2. Red-footed tortoise (*Geochelone carbonaria*) digestive tract (Stevens and Hume, 1995).

intestine allows for the greater digestion of the fibrous material they are eating, leading to a longer retention time. As tortoises are very important in seed dispersal in their native habitats, there has been much study in the field regarding retention rates. Red-footed tortoises were shown to have a retention rate of approximately 18.92 ± 4.81 days, with the sex of the animal being an important indicator of mean retention rate as females appear to have longer retention times than males.[6]

One of the factors to consider with digestion and retention time in captive animals is adequate heat sources for the turtles and tortoises. As ectotherms, these animals require an external heat source to properly digest their food. For turtles, this means their water should be heated to between 68 and 82°F depending on the species, and the enclosure should contain an adequate basking spot on dry land that allows the turtle bask in a temperature between 85 and 95°F. The area should also be large enough to allow them to move in and out of "hot spots." Tortoises should also be provided a basking area within the same temperature. If possible, the animals should have access to unfiltered natural sunlight to facilitate their own Vitamin D_3 production in their skin, but if they are housed indoors, they will require a full-spectrum ultraviolet-B (UVB) basking lamp with an exposure time of 20 to 30 min periods 2 to 3 times weekly.

Defecation and urination both occur from the cloacal opening also known as the vent. Although retention times of the food may be long in some animals, most adult turtles and tortoises will defecate every 2 to 4 days. Younger animals should defecate daily, but as they mature, this time will increase. This timeframe is a loose one, and actual defecation rates will vary by species, size, and sex of animals, with larger animals defecating less often, and generally males defecating more often than females. If an adult animal is defecating daily or less than once a week, this could be an indication that something is wrong and that intervention may be necessary. It helps to know the animals in your care and get a feel of what their normal defecation patterns. Defecation in tortoises can be stimulated through warm water baths that are between 95 and 105°F. Tortoises need to be soaked 1-2X weekly for at least 20 min. to keep them hydrated, for the health of their skin, and to help with defecation.

The size, color, and texture of the feces will depend on the animal's diet. Turtles have smaller round feces that do not disintegrate in water, and terrestrial species will have more fibrous green or brown feces, but they should be well-shaped. There is an excellent red-footed tortoise fecal scoring chart that can be accessed at the AZA Nutritional Advisory Group website.[7] Along with feces, they will urinate out uric acid. In aquatic turtles, this uric acid is more dilute, so their it will come out clear. In terrestrial turtles and tortoises, the uric acid is more concentrated, and it will dry into what is known as urate which will generally have a white milky appearance when it is first eliminated which dries into a chalky white hard powder.

Growth
Growth rate at a young age is very important for these animals. Diets with a lower protein to fat ratio will lead to rapid growth in body mass without the concomitant increase

Table 1
Growth data for head-started Western Pond Turtles (*Acitinemys marmorata*) at the Oregon Zoo from 2006 to 2016

Cohort Year	Capture Date	Release Dates	n	Initial Wt (g)	Last Wt (g)	Gain (g)	Days Head-Started (d)	Growth Rate (g/d)
2006[a]	Sept 2006	Aug 2007	47	5.3	82.9	77.6	322	0.24
2007[a]	Sept 2007	Jul 2008	55	5.5	82.7	77.2	324	0.24
2008[a]	Sept 2008	Jul 2009	53	5.7	108.3	102.7	312	0.33
2009[b]	Sept 2009	Jul 2010	63	5.3	133.3	128.0	315	0.41
2010[b]	Sept 2010	Jul/Aug 2011	40	5.3	150.9	145.6	308	0.47
2011[b]	May/Jun 2011	Jun 2012	18	6.8	161.7	154.9	378	0.41
2011[b]	Sept/Oct 2011	Jul 2012	27	6.1	131.7	125.6	310	0.41
2012[b]	Sept 2012	Jun 2013	11	6.4	153.0	146.6	278	0.53
2012[b]	May 2012	Jun 2013	15	6.8	181.4	174.6	403	0.43
2012[b]	Sept 2012	Aug 2012	8	6.1	128.1	122.0	319	0.38
2016[c]	Apr/May 2016	Oct 2016	6	6.1	42.9	36.9	153	0.25
2016[c]	Apr/May 2016	Jul/Aug 2017	14	6.5	54.1	46.3	362	0.13

[a] Diet: Unknown.
[b] Diet: Herring, Nightcrawlers, Pinkie Mice, Waxworms, Mealworms (5.28 kcal/g, 56.8% CP, 33.7% Fat, 1.36% Ca, 1.49% P, 0.91 Ca:P Ratio.
[c] Diet: Commercial Aquatic Turtle Pelleted Diet, Commercial Aquatic Turtle Gel, Lake Smelt, Nightcrawlers, Mealworms (3.89 kcal/g, 44.8% CP, 12.2% Fat, 2.0% Ca, 1.5% P, 1.41 Ca:P Ratio).

in bone and shell growth. This can tend to lead to obesity and weak bones and set animals up for susceptibility conditions such as metabolic bone disease.

The Western Pond Turtle is an endangered species in the Pacific Northwest due to predation by invasive bullfrog populations. Conservation efforts have been in place for decades that bring eggs and hatchling turtles into captivity and raise them until they are at a size beyond predation by bullfrogs. **Table 1** summarizes different cohorts raised over the years in one institution. When the program started, the growth rate was approximately 0.24 g/d. Observations from keepers at the time indicated the diet was as natural as possible, but, as the years continued, diet items that were higher in fat started to be substituted due to animal preference. The diet rose to an energy level of 5.28 kcal/g, 56.8% CP, 33.7% Fat, and the Ca:P ratio fell to 0.91. In just 6 years' time, the growth rate grew to up to 0.53 g/d, which was more than twice the rate measured at the beginning of the program. Animals were more than double the size of cohorts from previous years even when being fed for similar amounts of time. Adjustments of the diets to remove fattier items and implementation of commercial pelleted and gel diets helped to lower the growth rate to a more natural level and improve the Ca:P ratio. The resulting diet of 3.89 kcal/g, 44.8% CP, 12.2% Fat, and a Ca:P ratio of 1.41 was able to reestablish the growth rate to <0.30 g/d.

In a review of freshwater turtle nutrition by Rawski and colleagues, they gathered data from studies with Chinese softshell turtles (*Pelodiscus sinensis*), which is a farmed species in China.[8] They concluded that the optimum level for young turtles was 39.0 to 46.5% CP and 8.8% fat with a 2:1 Ca:P ratio.

Conversely, Avery and colleagues found that lower protein levels led to suboptimal growth rates, and that levels between 25 and 40% CP were required to optimize the growth of both shell length and body mass of juvenile slider turtles.[9] They determined that a carnivorous or omnivorous diet may require a significant amount of fish or other animal protein to sustain the high juvenile growth rates. Further, the adults of the species have a diet consisting of almost entirely vegetation.

Together from these observations, one can determine that a minimal amount of protein needed for turtles for optimal growth would be 25%; however, optimal growth would likely be >45% and <55% CP, but this would also require a dietary fat level of less than 15% to prevent rapid growth and possible obesity.

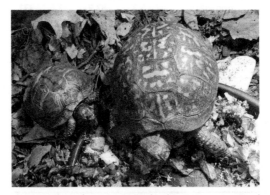

Fig. 3. Two Eastern box turtles of approximately the same age. Turtle on the right was brought in as an injured rescue from the wild. Turtle on the left was brought in after being kept as a personal pet and fed an unbalanced diet that consisted mainly of a commercial dog food. Notice the smaller relative size, the severe pyramiding on the shell, and the malformed beak, when compared to the turtle on the right. (Photo credit: Matt Brooks.)

Several commercial turtle diets are formulated at CP levels of 35 to 40% CP and 6 to 10% Fat. These diets area also formulated with a Ca:P ratio between 1.5 and 2.0:1. When possible, veterinarians should be recommending the use of commercial diets that are properly formulated for turtle species. Clients should be advised against feeding diets formulated for other animals. As illustrated in **Fig. 3**, proper food selection and formulation can drastically affect growth of the animal. The turtle on the right was an injured turtle brought in to the rehabilitation facility from the wild, and the animal on the left in the picture was kept as a pet most of its life. Both box turtles in **Fig. 3** are of the same approximate age; however, the one on the left and is of a much smaller size due to being fed a commercial kibble dog food diet at a young age. Even assuming a higher quality puppy food diet designed with higher protein is still only approximately 21 to 28% protein, and it has an increased fat level of 15 to 18%. The Ca:P ratio of dog or cat food diets is usually formulated to around 1.0 to 1.2. This makes this an inadequate diet for feeding turtles at any stage of life.

Tortoises have evolved to subsist on vegetation which has a lower energy and protein level that animal-based food items. These low energy and protein and high fiber density food plants are digested slowly in the hind-gut of the animal, and this allows for maximal absorption to provide more energy from these lower quality feeds. Hazard and colleagues fed juvenile desert tortoises different diets of either grasses or forbes and found that the diets containing between 18 to 26% CP and 19 to 37% Fiber produced positive growth in the growing tortoises, while diets that were strictly grass and contained 4 to 5% CP and 49 to 50% Fiber were inadequate for growth and led to weight loss in the animals.[10] The animals fed the inadequate diet lost body mass and shell volume on these diets. As turtles mature, the amount of dietary protein required for maintenance decreases, allowing adult turtles to subsist on diets as low as 10 to 12% CP. As mentioned previously, excess protein and energy can lead to malformations and weak bones. In tortoises, excess protein has been shown to cause soft shell (osteomalacia) and uricacidaemia.[11–13] Know that when feeding growing tortoises, a slightly higher CP level is required between the 18 to 26% range, and as they mature, the CP range can decrease to 8 to 12% CP.

Commercial tortoise diets are now being formulated with less starch to reduce the rapidly digestible energy source. These diets can be found that are formulated for smaller growing tortoises and larger mature tortoises with the aforementioned CP levels.

The best recommendation that can be given to any animal caretaker is to buy a scale and weigh the animals regularly. Accurate and consistent record keeping, even for a household with a pet turtle, is going to be the best way to determine if the animal is growing at a proper rate.

Body Condition Scoring

Body condition scoring is a method to assess an animal's fitness that goes beyond just weight. This method takes into account the animal's frame size and muscle mass and is a way to give a quantitative measure to a qualitative assessment. It is a way to evaluate the amount of muscle tone and fat stores of an animal to determine if the animal is under- or over-nourished for its body size. These Body Condition Scores (BCS) are generally a numerical scale. Initially, the scales started as a 1 to 5 scale, but the more accurate and preferred scale has become a 1 to 9 scale. Generally, the rankings for a 1 to 9 scale are: 1 to 3 – Under-condition; 4 to 6 – Acceptable or Good Condition; 7 to 9 Over-condition. Many of these scales have even been verified through post-mortem evaluation and ultrasonography. Although many people may be familiar with the BCS charts of dogs and cats, there have been BCS charts produced for animals all across the animal kingdom from elephants and eagle rays to sandhill cranes and spiders. The AZA Nutritional Advisory Group website (NAGOnline.net) has compiled as many of the known BCS charts as possible in the Body Condition Score Resource Center to provide as an online resource for all users.

Each animal can provide its own challenges. For many mammals, a thick fur coat can make a visual assessment almost impossible. For birds, it is trying to assess the shape of the body on the keel to determine if there is more muscle or fat. As one can imagine, shelled animals provide a very unique complication in that their soft tissues are mostly contained in a hard outer shell. Rawski and Józefiak do an excellent job of outlining what is necessary to produce a BCS system for the African side-neck turtle.[14] It requires creating models for the scale that provide a visual range from thin to obese animals to outline areas on the animals that will best assess body composition through visualization and palpation. For turtles, tortoises and other reptiles, a large portion of their adipose tissue accumulates in the subcutaneous areas. In shelled animals, the best areas for assessment are around the legs and can be very telling when an animal pulls itself into its shell and either cannot pull its limb or head properly into its shell, or when it does pull its limbs in, rolls of fat protrude out from shell. **Fig. 4** highlights the contrasts between an African snake-necked turtle in a healthy body condition score of a 4 out of a scale of 9 (see **Fig. 4**A) and an obese turtle 8 out of a scale of 9 (see **Fig. 4**B) that has so much excess fat that it can barely pull its rear limbs under its shell.

There have been more in-depth charts created for desert tortoises and Greek tortoises.[15,16] The scoring system for the desert tortoises goes beyond just subcutaneous fat store assessment and assesses the feel of the tortoise by weight, muscle mass, and concave or convex assessment on the limbs and top of the head, while also looking at the subcutaneous fat on the cervical, axillary, and inguinal regions of the tortoise. The article by Lamberski has multiple pictures from multiple angles to help get the best visual picture possible of the tortoises' physical state.[15] Willemsen and Hailey have a more quantitative measure of body condition by looking at the

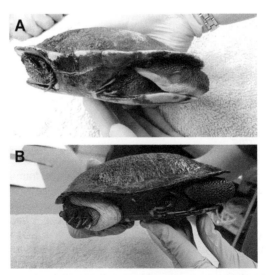

Fig. 4. (*A*) Lateral view of an Australian snake-necked turtle (*Chelodina longicollis*) in good body condition (4/9 scale). (*B*) Lateral view of an Australian snake-necked turtle (*Chelodina longicollis*) in poor body condition (8/9 scale). (Photo credit: Matt Brooks.)

mass to length ratio to calculate a condition index (CI).[16] However, they noted that even though these CIs could be extrapolated out from one population to the next, they were species specific and could be affected by season and geographic location.

For practical purposes, the BCS system is a fast and efficient way to assess an animal, but it does require a practiced hand. The best way to learn how to assess BCS is to put eyes and hands on as many animals as possible. Take pictures of animals from multiple angles and compare photos of other animals of the same species to help with training yourself and others. Over time and practice, you will learn to determine what is fat and muscle and where to look and feel on a specific species to best assess their condition. Also, as mentioned earlier, continue to take regular weights of the animals in your care and compare these weights to body condition scores.

Diet items

For chelonians in human care, providing a "natural" or "wild" diet with exactitude is going to be very difficult to almost impossible if they are kept in areas outside of their native ranges, as many are. However, their nutritional needs can be met with a properly formulated diet. For the animals in human care, this is best met with a combination of raw foods and formulated commercial feeds.

Commercial diets

As mentioned previously, there are several commercial diets on the market that are formulated especially for turtles or tortoises. These diets are generally meant to be a "complete" diet, meaning they provide all the nutrients the animal needs without other diet items or supplementation. However, some diets are meant to be fed with other diet items, so it is always best to feed the diet as directed by the manufacturer.

Although commercial diets do not always make up a majority of the weight of the food being offered to the animal, they do make up the bulk of the nutrition for the animal. This is because they are a more nutrient dense diet item that contains most, if not all, the protein, fat, fiber, vitamins, and minerals that animal needs. They are the most important diet item in the diet of an animal in human care. If an animal is wild caught or has not been previously reared on these commercial diets, it can be sometimes be difficult to get them to accept these diets. This is also why these items come in multiple forms. Most are extruded pellets, but there are also gel diets available. The benefit of gel diets is the ability to add other diet items into the gel while it is being formed. Adding bits of fish or insects into the gel can make it more appealing for the turtles. This can also be used as a way of administering medications orally, if the animal will readily consume the gels in their entirety. For turtles, the pelleted and gel diets are generally designed to float on top of the water. For tortoises, the pelleted diets can be fed dry by themselves, they can be moistened with water or even dilute juice, or they can be mixed with the salad portion of the diet to help with acceptance. One method to help with consumption for animals that do not readily accept the pellets is to grind them up into a powder and mix them with fresh greens. Allowing them to sit for a short while in refrigeration with the greens will moisten the powder and it will "stick" to the greens so the animal will consume the formulated diet with every bite of their salad.

Invertebrates

For the omnivorous and carnivorous turtles, invertebrates in the diet are not only essential portions, they can also provide some feeding enrichment for the animal. Rawski and colleagues published a table with a list of whole prey fed to freshwater turtles.[8] This table can help provide guidance when selecting the best animal protein to feed to your turtles or omnivorous tortoises. These items are high in protein (31–81% CP), but the items that are higher in fat should be limited to being rarely or never fed.

Items such as wax moth larva or neonatal mice are not only low in protein and high in fat, they are also deficient in other vital nutrients such as Ca and vitamin A. To the turtles, these are the equivalent of feeding them candy, and to their determinant, they will usually stop eating other portions of their diet in favor of these high-fat items. It is recommended to reserve these items to be fed as vehicles for medication. Commercially available insects are also generally lower in Ca and higher in P, leading to an inverse Ca:P ratio (<1.0:1). Crickets, for example, can have Ca:P ratio of 0.15:1, which is well below the desired 1.5 to 2:1. To combat this, insects such as mealworms and crickets can be "gut-loaded," which is the process of feeding the insect a diet high in calcium within 24 hours of feeding them to the turtle. In this way, the higher calcium gut contents of the insect will be fully consumed with the insect. Given the correct insect gut-loading diet, crickets can reach a 1:1 or 1.5:1 Ca:P ratio. There are some invertebrates of note that are naturally higher in their Ca:P ratios. These include nightcrawlers and dried black soldier fly larva. These make excellent choices when putting together a diet for a turtle or omnivorous tortoise.

Vertebrates

Vertebrate animals are items regularly fed to growing and turtles and the more carnivorous adult turtles. Fish especially can be a major portion of the diet for many animals. Snapping turtles in particular subsist mainly on fish in their diet. For freshwater turtles, it is best to feed them freshwater fish species, as salt-water species will have a salt content that could not be good to the animal. If salt-water species are the only option available, the thawed fish can be soaked in water prior to feeding to help leach out the salt content of the fish before feeding. This should be done using safe food handling practices under refrigeration, and the water can be replaced multiple times to help remove as much salt as possible. Some fish also contain an enzyme known as thiaminase and high levels of polyunsaturated acids. When fish are frozen, these reduce the levels of thiamin and vitamin E the longer they sit in the freezer. Fish such as goldfish, smelt, and minnows, which are the most commercially available fish, can end up being deficient in these two nutrients. If these fish are a major portion of a turtle's diet, it is recommended to supplement the animals either orally or parenterally with 25 mg thiamin/kg body weight and 1 IU vitamin E/kg body weight.[17] Mice and day-old chickens are other items that can be used. For smaller turtles, these items would need to be cut into pieces before being fed.

Produce

Chelonians consume a myriad of vegetation in the wild. Their varied diet helps to make sure their diet in the wild stays nutritionally complete. In managed care, the variety of commercially available produce is diminished in comparison. The choice of produce to purchase when shopping for your turtle or tortoise needs to be carefully considered due to several nutritional factors inherent in the items available. Some things to watch out for when selecting produce include the nutrient density, mineral content, and the levels of certain secondary plant compounds. Iceberg lettuce is an example of produce that is not nutrient dense. The water content of this lettuce is so high that it is not going to provide a lot of nutrition in the diet and should be avoided in favor of other lettuces such as romaine, green/red leaf, or butter lettuce. The level of calcium and phosphorous should be considered when picking produce such as dark leafy greens. Dandelion greens and romaine lettuce have a Ca:P ratio of 2.8 to 3:1, which makes them excellent choices for greens.[17] Some secondary plant compounds to avoid at high levels are oxalates/oxalic acid, which are compounds that bind up calcium in the gut and prevent absorption.[18] Spinach and Red/Swiss Chard are very high in oxalates and should be avoided as regular diet items. Goitrogens are another second-ary plant compound to avoid. They interfere with the utilization of iodine in the body and lead to an enlargement of the thyroid gland. These can be found in cruciferous vegetables.[18] It is hard to find some of the green vegetables that do not contain some level of these compounds. This makes it crucial that a diet does not rely on one particular type of vegetable all the time. Using a variety of produce items helps mitigate the higher levels of these compounds in certain produce items. There are no exhaustive lists of safe vs unsafe produce for turtles and tortoises. It is best to eval-uate each produce choice one-by-one to determine if it something that should be fed to a chelonian or not.

Supplementation

Most captive diets require some sort of supplementation with vitamins and minerals to ensure it is a complete diet. In the wild, the animals would be ingesting diet items with better nutritional profiles than what is available commercially, as discussed above. They would also be getting passive ingestion of minerals from the soils and water on/in which they eat. As the captive environment is arguably more "nutritionally ster-ile," the best practice is to supplement the animals with a commercial product designed for their unique needs. Without sufficient levels of calcium in the diet, their body stores will be depleted, their shells will not calcify properly, and they will develop metabolic bone disease.[19,20] Providing a cuttlebone in the animal's enclosure is a good source of calcium that is also useful for wearing down their beak. There are a variety of commercially available supplements for reptiles. The important items to look for in a supplement are the calcium, phosphorus, and vitamin A concentration. The other vitamin that needs to be considered is Vitamin D_3, which is required for proper calcium metabolism. If an animal is diurnal (active during the day) and is outside or under UVB lamps, then extra dietary Vitamin D_3 supplementation is likely unneces-sary. However, if the animal is nocturnal, or is diurnal and kept indoors away from ac-cess to UVB lighting, then supplemental D_3 is necessary. There are currently products marketed today with and without additional vitamin D_3. As concentrations for these products can vary, the amount to feed should be based on the manufacturer's recom-mendation for their product.

Sample diets

First, it should be noted that the recommendations in this section are made in the form of percentages of groups of diet items that are in the diet. However, the amounts fed to the specific animal will need to be determined on an individual basis. To do this re-quires assessing the species, the life stage (juvenile, adult, breeding, and so forth), environment, seasonal patterns, and activity level. The best tool to help with monitor how the animal is responding to all of these factors is through quantitative assessment through body condition scoring, tracking weight, and tracking the amount of food the animal consumes and leaves with each feeding. This is why it is critical to use a scale to weigh and record not only the animal, but the food fed out and the food refused (orts). Changes in food consumption outside of normal seasonal patterns is one of the first indicators of something wrong in the animal.

This leads into the question of feeding frequency. Many caretakers want to know if they should feed their animal every day, every other day, or provide a fast day. For most reptiles, they do not need to eat every day. Animals that are more active, such as the freshwater turtles, will do well being fed every day as long as quantities are con-trol. Adding fast days, in the week can be beneficial in a couple of ways. First, the an-imal will likely do better about maintaining weight. Turtles and tortoises can gain

Table 2
Sample diets, by percentage (%), fed to different species of turtles in human care

			Freshwater Turtle			Terrestrial Turtles
	WPT[a] Juvenile[b]	WPT[a] Adult[c]	Slider/Painted	Snake-Necked	Giant Pond/Arrua River	Eastern/Ornate Box
Aquatic Turtle Pelleted Diet	45	25	4	33		
Aquatic Carnivorous Reptile Gel	22	19				
Aquatic Herbivorous Turtle Gel					50	
Tortoise Low-starch Pelleted Diet						3
Annelids	11	6	11	33		7
Insects	6	8				1
Fish	11	11	52	33		
Mammals	5					
Hardboiled Egg Whites						15
Dark Leafy Greens/Cabbages		31	33			40
Lettuce					10	
Broccoli						11
Root Vegetables					10	10
Squashes					20	
Cucumber/Zucchini					10	
Fruit						13

[a] Western Pond Turtle.
[b] Juvenile for this species is any turtle weighing between 6 and 63 g.
[c] Adult for this species is any turtle weighing > 350g.

Table 3
Sample diets, by percentage (%), fed to different species of tortoises in human care

| | Omnivorous Tortoise | Herbivorous Tortoises | | | |
	Red-Footed	African Spurred	Desert/ Leopard	Egyptian/Pancake/ Radiated/Spider	Russian
Tortoise Low-starch Pelleted Diet	20	24	40	3	10
Hardboiled Egg Whites	2				
Dark Leafy Greens/Cabbages	39	38	40	65	60
Broccoli	10	20	10	17	15
Root Vegetables	17	13	10	15	15
Fruit	12	5	<1%		<1%
Hay	Ad Libitum	Ad Libitum	Ad Libitum	Ad Libitum	-

weight very easily, so controlling intake and digestion time with fast days can help with this. Second, if an animal is being picky about certain diet items, they are more likely to accept these less than desired items on the day after a fast day. The best example of this is when an animal does not want to eat the commercial diet. If this is the case, feed the commercial diet as the first meal after a fast day. As an animal gets older and passes out of the rapid growth phase, fast days can become a regular part of the weekly routine. There are times of the year when a turtle or tortoise's appetite is elevated, and fast days may not be necessary; for example, breeding season for females or when a turtle or tortoise has just come out of brumation.

For young freshwater turtles that are mostly carnivorous from hatch until maturation a suggested diet would be to use a diet that is about 50% commercial food and 50% protein sources including invertebrates, mammals, and fish. **Table 2** shows an example diet for hatchling Western Pond turtles (*Actinemys marmorata*) that weigh between 6.0 and 63.0g. In contrast, **Table 3** shows an example diet for adults (>350 g body weight) of the same species. The adult diet is approximate 45% formulated commercial diet, 30% greens, and 25% protein sources from invertebrates and fish. This diet is not set in stone for all omnivorous turtles, as some tend more toward carnivory even in adult life. The painted turtles and sliders can have fewer pellets if provided with adequate amounts of fish, but they still need to have the pelleted diet to ensure they are getting their necessary levels of vitamins and minerals. The Australian snake-necked turtle is an example of a fully carnivorous turtle that does not eat any produce, while the Giant Malaysian Pond and Arrua river turtles opportunistically omnivorous in the wild feeding on fruit and other vegetations that falls into the ponds and streams they inhabit; however, they have been also observed to eat fish. Little is known of the actual amount of herbivory vs carnivory, but fecal samples and anecdotal evidence would suggest that they are primarily herbivorous animals.[1]

The terrestrial turtles have one of the widest arrays of possible diet items available (see **Table 2**). They are able to eat just about anything they come across in the wild. Part of this strategy is likely the way they meet all their nutritional needs when it comes to vitamins and minerals.[21] This is also one of the reasons that very little of the commercial diet is necessary in the diet. This diet focuses heavily on the root vegetables (10%) and leafy greens (40%) with supplemental protein from eggs (15%) and invertebrates (11%). These turtles can also tolerate more fruit (13%) in their diet than other chelonians, as they opportunistically will eat fallen fruit in the forests they inhabit. That being said, the level of fruit should not exceed 15% of their diet, or it could lead to digestive issues and diarrhea.

The diets used for tortoises (see **Table 3**) are very similar in composition because the diets consist mostly of a commercial diet and produce. The exception in the provided examples are found in the diet of the omnivorous tortoises such as the red-footed tortoise. These animals, such as the terrestrial turtles whose diet is shown in **Table 2**, have a higher protein requirement, and they can tolerate a higher sugar content, so they can have diet items such as hardboiled egg whites and higher levels of fruit. Many species of tortoises should also have hay provided *ad libitum*, as it is their major fiber source. As there are always exceptions, there are some tortoises, such as the Russian tortoise, that are not grass eaters, so they do not eat hay, but they will consume dried edible flowers.

Future Direction

The difficulty with coming up with recommendations for turtles and tortoises is the lack of formal study that has been applied to the nutrition of this vast family of reptiles. This area is a veritable "gold mine" of information that could be had if given its proper due. In fact, much of the information that has been applied in the field thus far to the husbandry and rearing of turtles and tortoises has come from the hobbyists who spend countless hours working with their particular animals in looking at food, habitat, reproduction, and health. Those among us in the academic field would do well to make more use of a collaboration with the hobbyists to provide more scientific rigor to the work they are already preforming.

SUMMARY

Caring for chelonians is a deeply rewarding endeavor, but it is one that takes a great deal of research when it comes to their nutritional health. These animals can live very long lives if they are cared for properly by putting proper attention into their diet, growth, and eating habits. It is important to make sure to consider that not all chelonians are the same, and diets and feeding regimes should be tailored to match the feeding ecology of the species of interest, whether it dwell in water or on land. Using this starting point, it then becomes matter of choosing food items that will garner the proper protein, fat, and energy balance needed for the chelonians stage of life. Once the diet is selected, it is a matter of constant, careful monitoring of the animal's eating habits, defecation routine, and body condition as ways to monitor animal health and adjust as necessary.

CLINICS CARE POINTS

- Imbalances in crude protein can lead to an unnatural acceleration or retardation of growth. Turtles and tortoises each have unique feeding strategies that require different levels of energy and protein to ensure they are meeting, but not exceeding, their growth potential.
- The Ca:P ratio needs to be between 1:4 and 2:0 for proper growth of chelonian's shell and bones.
- The best ways to monitor your animal's nutritional health is to weigh them regularly, weigh the food they consume, and to practice body condition scoring them to ensure they are not getting too thin or too heavy.

> • Make sure the diet items and proportions are appropriate for the type of turtle or tortoise you are feeding. Use the provided sample diets as a base to help craft an appropriate diet.

REFERENCES

1. Kimmel CE. A diet and reproductive study for selected species of Malaysian turtles. Masters Thesis. Charleston, IL: Eastern Illinois University; 1980.
2. Donaldson BM, Echternacht AC. Aquatic habitat use relative to home range and seasonal movement of Eastern box turtles (*Terrapene carolina carolina*: Emydidae) in Eastern Tennessee. J Herp 2005;39(2):284–7.
3. Coe MJ, Bourn D, Swingland IR. The biomass, production, and carrying capacity of giant tortoises on Aldabra. Phil Trans R Soc Lond 1979;286:163–76.
4. Bouchard SS, Bjorndal KA. Nonadditive interactions between animal and plant diet items in an omnivorous freshwater turtle. Trachemys scripta. Comp Biochem Physiol Part B 2006;144:77–85.
5. Stevens CE, Hume ID. Comparative physiology of the vertebrate digestive system. 2nd edition. New York: Cambridge University Press; 1995.
6. Rodrigues LL, Souza Y, Galetti M. Frugivory and seed dispersal by the red-footed tortoise *Chelonoidis carbonaria*. Acta Oecol 2022;116(6):103837.
7. Mendoza P, Furuta C. Red-footed tortoise (Chelonoidis carbonaria) faecal scoring chart. In: AZA Nutrition Advisory Group Fecal Condition Scoring Resource Center. 2020. Available at: https://nagonline.net/wp-content/uploads/2018/04/Mendoza-and-Furuta-2020.png. Accessed June 13, 2023.
8. Rawski M, Mans C, Kierończyk B, et al. Freshwater turtle nutrition – A review of scientific and practical knowledge. Ann Anim Sci 2018;18(1):17–37.
9. Avery HW, Spotila JR, Congdon JD, Fisher RU Jr, et al. Roles of diet protein and temperature in the growth and nutritional energetics of juvenile slider turtles, *Trachemys scripta*. Physiol Zoo 1993;66(6):863–1049.
10. Hazard LC, Shemanski DR, Nagy KA. Nutritional quality of natural foods of juvenile desert tortoises (*Gopherus agassizii*): Energy, nitrogen, and fiber digestibility. J Herp 2009;43(1):38–48.
11. Homer B, Berry K, Brown H, et al. Pathology of diseases in wild desert tortoises from California. J Wildl Dis 1998;34:508–23.
12. Scot PW. Nutritional diseases. In: Manual of reptiles, beynon, PH. Gloucestershire: British Small Animal Veterinary Association; 1992. p. 128–37.
13. Wronski TJ, Yen CF, Jacobson ER. Histomorphometric studies of dermal bone in the desert tortoise, *Gopherus agassizii*. J Wildl Dis 1992;28:603–9.
14. Rawski M, Józefiak D. Body condition scoring and obesity in captive African sideneck turtles (*Pelomedusidae*). Ann Anim Sci 2014;14(3):573–84.
15. Lamberski N. Body condition scores for desert tortoises. In: AZA Nutrition Advisory Group Body Condition Scoring Resource Center. 2011. Available at: https://nagonline.net/wp-content/uploads/2016/08/Desert-Tortoise.pdf. Accessed June 13, 2023.
16. Willemsen RE, Hailey A. Body mass condition in Greek tortoises: Regional and interspecific variation. Herp J 2002;12:105–14.
17. Donoghue S, McKeown S. Nutrition of captive reptiles. Vet Clinics N Amer: Exotic Anim Practice 1999;2(1):69–91.
18. Sinha K, Khare V. Review on: Antinutritional factors in vegetable crops. Pharma Innov J 2017;6(12):353–8.

19. Fledelius B, Jørgensen GW, Jensen HE, et al. Influence of calcium content of the diet offered to leopard tortoises (*Geochelone pardalis*). Vet Rec 2005;156:831–5.
20. Gerlach J. Effects of diet on the systemic utility of the tortoise carapace. African J Herpetol 2004;53(1):77–85.
21. Hailey A, Chidavaenzi RL, Loveridge JP. Diet mixing in the omnivorous tortoise *Kinixys spekii*. Func Ecol 1998;12:373–85.

Mini Pig Nutrition and Weight Management

Nichole F. Huntley, MS, PhD

KEYWORDS

- Mini pig • Potbelly pig • Nutrition • Feeding • Weight management

KEY POINTS

- Pigs are omnivores that naturally root and forage throughout the day. These behaviors must be considered when caring for and feeding mini pigs.
- Mini pigs easily gain weight. A balanced, high-fiber diet helps maintain healthy body condition, and body condition scoring is an essential tool for weight management.
- Published nutrient requirements for production pigs are a good reference but must be interpreted in the context of pet mini pigs, prioritizing longevity and healthy weight maintenance.

BACKGROUND

Miniature pig, or mini pig, is a broad, general category covering multiple breeds of domestic pigs (*Sus scrofa*) with a mature size relatively smaller than their full-sized production pig relatives. The Vietnamese potbellied pig was introduced into North America in the mid-1980s, originally intended for zoos, but it became a popular pet. Since then, efforts to develop smaller pet pigs coalesced with the development of miniature versions of swine biomedical research models leading to today's multiple varieties and breeds (a loosely used term).[1] In this article, "mini pig" encompasses potbellied pigs, American mini pigs, Juliana pigs, Kunekunes, Göttingen pigs, and any other smaller breeds maintained as pets.

Pigs are monogastric omnivores (**Fig. 1**) that evolved from wild boars, which forage on grasses, fruits, roots, and invertebrates.[2,3] They are curious animals with a strong motivation to root, forage, and explore their environment. This behavior must be a primary consideration when caring for and feeding mini pigs.

SCOPE OF THIS ARTICLE

There are many strong opinions among the mini-pig community. Blogs and social media groups are common places owners seek information; unfortunately, misinformation is

Mazuri Exotic Animal Nutrition, PMI Nutrition International, 4001 Lexington Avenue North, Arden Hills, MN 55126, USA
E-mail address: nhuntley@mazuri.com

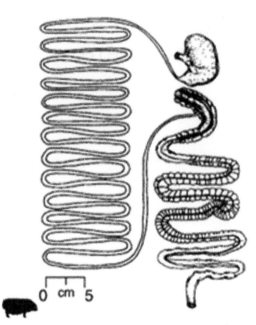

Fig. 1. Pig (Sus scrofa) digestive tract (from Stevens & Hume 1995[4]).

prevalent. However, there are many quality resources available. At the time of this publication, the most comprehensive is Potbellied Pig Veterinary Medicine by Kristie Mozzachio.[1] This article is intended to expand on currently available nutrition information with a focus on topics important for weight management.

NUTRIENT REQUIREMENTS

There are no definitive nutrient requirements determined specifically for mini pigs. Nutrient requirements are published in the Swine NRC[5] for production pigs fed ad libitum for efficient and rapid growth. Some research is also available for biomedical mini-pig models. These nutrient requirements likely apply to mini pigs[6] but must be critically evaluated in the context of mini pig growth curves and lifestyle goals, prioritizing longevity and healthy weight maintenance. To achieve these goals, mini pigs must be limit fed to prevent excessive weight gain (as much as 40%–60% of ad libitum intake is necessary to prevent obesity.[7,8]) Therefore, vitamins and minerals must be more concentrated, or evaluated on a total intake basis, in mini pig diets compared to NRC recommendations.[5]

Energy

Metabolizable energy (ME) requirements for maintenance have been published for laboratory mini pigs.[9] However, based on practical experience, these estimates are very high and would undoubtedly result in obesity of the typical pet mini pig. Swine NRC equations for maintenance energy requirements of growing pigs and sows[5] are more reasonable for calculating the daily caloric needs of mini pigs. However, it is necessary to note that these equations were developed for production pigs and should only be used as a starting point. Feed intake and calorie allotment should always be adjusted based on the individual pig's body condition and specific needs.

Resting energy requirements.

- Young, rapidly growing pigs[5]: kcal ME/day = 197 x (body weight in kg)$^{0.60}$
- Mini pigs at maintenance: kcal ME/day = 100 x (body weight in kg)$^{0.75}$
  - Based on the NRC for gestating sows but aligns with 40% to 60% restriction from ad libitum intake recommended for mini pigs.[7,8]
- Lactating sows[5]: kcal ME/d = 110 x (body weight in kg)$^{0.75}$

Daily energy requirements.

1. Using the equations above, apply a cofactor of 1.25 to 2.0 based on the pig's activity level. A cofactor of 1.0 should be used for weight loss.

Protein

Amino acids from protein are essential for proper growth and development, immune function, hormone production, digestion, and absorption, among many other biological functions. Total amino acid requirements and relative proportions depend on whole-body protein deposition in growing pigs and fetal growth rate lactation volume in sows. Chronic illness and injury recovery also change a pig's amino acid requirement.[5]

Feeding a diet specific to a pig's life stage is recommended. Too low of protein negatively impacts the growth and development of a young pig, while too much protein for a sedentary adult adds unnecessary strain on the kidneys. Up to 4 months of age, rapidly growing mini pigs should be fed a diet with at least 20% protein. After 4 months, pigs are still growing, though not as quickly, and should be fed a diet with about 16% protein. Active pigs can continue on a 14% - 16% protein diet until they are fully grown (between the ages of 3–5) or their activity level decreases and they start gaining excessive weight. At that point, mini pigs should be transitioned onto a lower protein (~12%) diet.

Fat

Dietary fat provides essential fatty acids, facilitates the absorption of fat-soluble vitamins, and is the most concentrated energy source in the diet. It is generally recommended to feed mini pigs diets with 3% to 4% fat.[1] Too much fat provides excessive calories, and too little may cause issues with dry, flaky skin – a common concern for mini pig owners.

The only published fatty acid requirement for pigs is linoleic acid (an omega-6 fatty acid), for which the swine NRC set at 0.10%.[5] As all animals do, pigs also require α-linolenic acid, an omega-3 fatty acid and metabolic precursor for eicosapentaenoic acid (EPA) and docosahexaenoic acid (DHA). Feed ingredients predominantly contain omega-6 fatty acids. However, a high omega-6-to-omega-3 ratio may contribute to excess inflammation in the body.[10] Therefore, it can be beneficial to feed diets enriched in omega-3 fatty acids, often provided by ingredients such as flaxseed and fish oil or from fresh grass.

Coconut oil, a source of medium-chain fatty acids such as lauric acid, is commonly supplemented to mini pigs due to the perceived health effects and improvement of skin dryness. Clinical evidence in humans supports the topical use of coconut oil to prevent and treat atopic dermatitis.[11] Although there is much anecdotal discussion about the benefits of coconut oil consumption, there is a lack of empirical data supporting this claim. For overweight pigs, coconut oil supplementation is not recommended due to its caloric density.

Vitamins and Minerals

The Swine NRC[5] vitamin and mineral requirements, expressed as an amount per day based on body weight, can be used as a guide for estimated mini pig daily vitamin and mineral requirements. Vitamins and minerals of particular interest for health issues commonly experienced by mini pigs are discussed in the relevant sections later in the discussion.

Water

Fresh water should be available to mini pigs at all times, but they are generally prandial drinkers.[1] Pigs are messy eaters and drinkers and often tip water bowls over if not secured. If this goes unnoticed, dehydration and salt toxicosis may occur. To prevent this, provide a bowl with a weighted bottom or wide base, secure the bowl within the center of a tire, or put the water in a container sunk into the ground so the pig cannot knock it over.

Fiber

There is no determined nutritional requirement for fiber in swine diets. However, there is no question that fiber is an essential component of a pig's diet, providing numerous benefits for their overall health and well-being (**Box 1**). Dietary fiber is defined as the non-digestible carbohydrates available for fermentation by intestinal microbiota. The mature pig's capacity for fiber fermentation and the amount of energy derived from the resulting short-chain fatty acids (SCFA) are often overlooked.

Fiber passes through the upper gastrointestinal tract (GIT) and is fermented by the anaerobic microbiota in the large intestine. Bacterial fermentation produces SCFA that can be absorbed and metabolized for energy. Mature and larger pigs have a greater fermentation capacity than younger and smaller pigs,[24] and SCFA can contribute more than 30% of the daily maintenance requirements for energy.[12] Short-chain fatty acids are a significant energy source for the epithelial lining of the GIT and help regulate host metabolism and the immune system.[25,26]

Fiber is classified according to its chemical constituents, physicochemical properties, and physiologic role in digestion. The primary categories relate to its solubility, viscosity - the ability to thicken or form gels in the GIT, and fermentability by the resident microbiota in the pig's hindgut. Generally, solubility correlates with viscosity, and all fibers fall somewhere on the gradients of soluble to insoluble and non-fermentable to 100% fermentable.

Soluble fiber is found in oats, barley, beet pulp, and some fruits and vegetables. Soluble and viscous fiber increase satiety by slowing gastric emptying, increasing the release of PYY and GLP-1, and attenuating post-prandial glycemic and insulinemic

---

Box 1
Fiber is an essential consideration in mini pig diets.

1. Fiber dilutes the calories of the pig's total diet.
   a. On average, a pig derives about 60% - 70% of the caloric value from fiber than sugar and starch carbohydrates,[12,13] and fiber decreases the energy digestibility of other ingredients in the feed.[12,14]

2. Fiber improves satiety by increasing gut fill and taking longer to digest.[15,16]
   a. This influences the production of gut hormones that promote satiety, such as glucagon-like peptide-1 (GLP-1) and peptide YY (PYY),[17] and reduces the frequency of hunger behaviors.[18-20]

3. Fiber supports gut health and, thus, pig health.[21,22]
   a. Fiber is a prebiotic that encourages the proliferation and maintenance of necessary commensal bacteria and discourages colonization by pathogenic bacteria.[23]

responses.[17,27] Most soluble fibers are moderately or highly fermentable and are pre-biotic substrates for microbial fermentation and SCFA production, which improve in-testinal health.[28] Sources of insoluble fiber for pigs include wheat bran, corn bran, soybean hulls, oat hulls, hay, and grass. Insoluble fiber increases fecal bulk and de-creases intestinal transit time, which supports regular bowel movements. Insoluble fi-ber is much less fermentable than soluble fiber, so fewer calories are derived from SCFA and the caloric density of the diet is decreased.

A balanced diet for pigs includes a mix of moderately fermentable, soluble, and insoluble fiber to optimize digestive health and overall well-being.[29,30] There is not enough research yet in companion pigs to specify an optimal soluble-to-insoluble ratio for mini pigs. However, based on studies in commercial pigs and other monogastric omnivores, a reasonable estimate is 3 - 4: 1, insoluble: soluble fiber.[12,27]

There are many methods by which fiber is analyzed and reported, and understand-ing the fundamental differences and applicability of each analysis is helpful for accu-rately assessing the fiber level in a pig's diet. References are available to understand which carbohydrate components each analysis determines and the completeness or reliability of each assay for its designated carbohydrate fraction.[31] The critical point is that there are different analyses which each give a very different picture of dietary fiber.

FEEDING RECOMMENDATIONS

A fortified, pelleted feed formulated specifically for mini pigs should constitute the base of the diet. Depending on the formulation, pellets should be at least 60% (dry matter basis) of a mature mini pig's total food intake, and 80% of a young growing pig's diet, to meet amino acid, vitamin, and mineral requirements. The remainder of the diet should consist of primarily non-starchy vegetables, leafy greens, and good-quality grass hay if they eat it (most, but not all, pigs will) or grass from grazing.

Pellets

Select a complete feed based on the pig's life stage and activity level. Mini pig specific feeds should be formulated to promote health and longevity and allow other food items to be incorporated. Commercial pig feed is intended for very different purposes: fast growth and efficient body weight gain (grower and finisher type diets) or to support the high nutrient requirements and high feed intake of a large sow during gestation and lactation. It is generally more calorically dense and often causes excessive weight gain in mini and potbelly pigs. Also, because most production pigs are fed ad libitum, commercial-type diets have lower concentrations of vitamins and minerals.

Produce

Mini-pig owners frequently implement elaborate meal plans, including daily salads. Produce is a great source of variety, and the high water content decreases the caloric density of the pig's diet and promotes hydration. Additionally, leafy greens and non-starchy vegetables are good fiber sources. It is essential to ensure that too much pro-duce is not fed so that the nutrients provided by the pellets are not diluted or unbalanced.

Although most pet pig owners prefer feeding nutritionally complete commercial pel-lets as the base of the diet, some are interested in feeding only produce and home-made food. This is frequently referred to as a "natural diet." However, food items consumed by wild pigs are substantially different nutritionally from the greens, vege-tables, and fruits cultivated for human consumption.[32,33] While a nutritionally balanced diet can be achieved through proper formulation and a very wide variety of food items, it is an unobtainable goal for most mini pig owners.

Homemade diets for pets have been consistently found to have at least one nutrient that was deficient and several that were out of balance in over 90% of 1,000s of diets analyzed.[34–37] Establishing a well-balanced homemade diet requires a complete understanding of the animal's nutritional requirements and the chemical composition and variability of all ingredients. Furthermore, a deep nutrition formulation understanding is necessary to combine foods in the right amounts and ratios to provide the pig with a well-balanced diet meeting all nutrient requirements. The nutritional adequacy of homemade diets also depends on the owner's ability to follow the recommended recipe strictly. They cannot always evaluate the effect of recipe deviations on the final nutritional composition and a nutrient deficiency or imbalance is often the result.[36]

Roughage

Roughage, such as hay and grass, is a significant source of fiber in a pig's diet, takes longer to eat, and encourages natural foraging and grazing behaviors. The extent to which roughage can contribute to the nutrient needs of pigs depends on the grass type and availability. If kept in the same pen where grass is initially available, pigs will quickly remove it, leaving overturned and bare earth. However, if you rotate areas or have sufficient space to maintain a grass stand, pigs can derive a significant amount of calories from grazing.[38] When pasture is not available, hay can be an excellent way to keep a pig occupied and satisfy their natural grazing behaviors. High-quality grass hays are preferred, and alfalfa should be avoided due to the higher protein, calorie, and calcium content.

Treats and Supplements

Fruit, cereal, oatmeal, unsalted popcorn, and commercially available mini pig treats are commonly fed items that should be used sparingly and strategically for training and behavior modification. Pigs are very food motivated, and a single small treat can go a long way. Lower-sugar and high-water content fresh fruits such as raspberries, strawberries, blackberries, or watermelon can be used for high-value rewards. Frozen coconut oil is commonly used as a treat or supplement, but even a small amount provides many calories due to its high fat content.

Many mini pig owners provide one or more supplements regularly. Common supplements include vitamin E, selenium, coconut oil, fish oil, biotin, and joint supplements. During a diet review, it is often necessary to ask specifically about treats and supplements since these are not always considered part of the pig's diet but contribute substantially to caloric and nutrient intake.

FEED ACCORDING TO LIFE STAGE
Juvenile

For young mini pigs, providing proper levels of protein and energy is essential to ensure healthy growth and development. Up to 4 months of age, feed a diet with 20% protein and easily digestible ingredients. Their digestive tracts are still geared toward digesting milk proteins and lactose, so it is important that high-quality, milk-derived ingredients, like whey, are included in the diet to help them transition easily from digesting milk to solid foods.

Creep feeding is a practice of providing highly digestible feed in a way that only the piglets can access to introduce the piglets to solid feed prior to weaning. Start with offering tiny amounts of pellets while piglets are still nursing, as early as 1-week post-farrowing. Feed small amounts frequently when the sow is eating or occupied. Initially, it is best to moisten the pellets, ideally with the sow's milk, to provide a gruel. Gradually the pellets should be moistened less and less so piglets are well adapted to eating dry pellets before weaning around 7 weeks of age. Young mini pigs do best with multiple feedings since their stomach is small and cannot fit much feed.

Adults

Mini pigs mature relatively quickly, so around 4 months old their growth rate changes but they are still growing and active. At this time, a mid-level protein diet is recommen-ded – around 16% protein, with more fiber starting to be incorporated. Miniature pigs generally reach half their adult weight by about 1 year and will continue to grow slowly until 3 to 5 years, when their growth plates fuse. Around 1 ½ years of age growth may start to slow down, so between the ages of 1 ½ and 3, depending on the body condi-tion and activity level, mini pigs living indoors who are less active should be transi-tioned to a maintenance-type diet with higher fiber and lower protein to help prevent excessive weight gain.

Reproduction

Pregnant females can be fed standard maintenance diets until the last few weeks of gestation, depending on their body condition. Around day 90 of gestation, calorie and protein requirements begin to increase. The sow should be transitioned onto a higher protein diet, and the total volume fed should be gradually increased. Under or overfeeding a pregnant or lactating sow can lead to problems with parturition, lacta-tion, and sow or piglet health,[39] so maintaining a healthy body condition is important.

The transition period of the last 10 days of gestation and the first 10 days of lactation brings a rapid shift in nutrient requirements due to an exponential increase in fetal and mammary growth, colostrum synthesis, and peak milk production.[40] Sows should be transitioned onto a higher protein and more calorically dense diet during that transition period and as long as necessary during lactation to maintain body condition. This can be achieved by mixing adult mini-pig food with feed for young, growing piglets. Due to the greater volume of food, feed 3 or more meals daily. Fresh water should always be available for the piglets and the sow, who drinks large volumes of water to support lactation. After weaning, the sow should return to her normal maintenance diet.

Geriatrics

The average lifespan of a mini pig is 12 to 15 years, but some live up to 18 to 20 years. As with all animals, providing good nutrition, plenty of exercise, and maintaining a healthy weight can help prolong the pig's lifespan. Chronic arthritis, secondary to poor hoof care or obesity, is a common reason for geriatric mini pigs to be euthanized, so good weight management and proper hoof care are key to longevity in mini pigs. Older mini pigs should continue to be fed a maintenance-type diet with a relatively low protein level (around 12%). If dentition is poor, moistening the feed with water can help improve consumption.

How Much to Feed

Like their larger production counterparts, mini pigs are highly efficient and easily gain excessive weight, and should never be fed free choice. A rule of thumb to determine how much to feed is based on body weight. For pigs 4 months old and younger, it is recommended that a mini pig consume 1.5% to 3% of body weight, in the total amount of food per day on an as-fed basis. For pigs older than 4 months, feed 1% to 2% of body weight, including all pellets, produce, roughage, and treats. The more active the pig, the higher in the range they should be fed. If a pig is overweight, its total food intake should be determined based on its estimated healthy weight rather than its current weight.

Refer to the manufacturer's feeding directions to determine what portion of the pig's total food intake must be pellets to meet the pig's nutrient requirements. Generally, a fortified pelleted feed should be at least 60% - 75% of the diet on a dry matter basis (25% - 40% on an as-fed basis due to the high moisture content of produce). Ideally, all food would be weighed out. However, that rarely happens, so cup measurements are most practical. Generally, one cup of mini pig pellets weighs 150 to 180 g, but a "cup" can refer to various volumes. So, when collecting diet history from mini pig owners, it is essential to clarify what a "cup" is in their household.

HEALTHY WEIGHT MANAGEMENT

Obesity is the number one health problem in pet pigs. If excessive weight is not addressed quickly, it can be challenging to improve. Obese pigs develop excessive fat around their face, hindering their ability to see and hear, and mobility is significantly reduced. Like other species, obesity increases the risk of metabolic and joint diseases and is associated with reduced longevity.[41–43] Obesity decreases an animal's quality of life, and successful weight loss is associated with improved welfare and quality of life.[44]

Body Condition Scoring

Pigs come in all shapes and sizes, so there is no "ideal weight" for mini pigs at different ages. This is why routinely evaluating and tracking their body condition is very important and is the best tool available to help maintain mini pigs at healthy weights. Body condition scoring (BCS) is a quantitative yet subjective management tool for evaluating body fat. Veterinarians and owners can use BCS to assess pigs of all ages and breeds, and it is a valuable diagnostic tool for managing weight loss and maintaining a healthy weight.

The American Mini Pig Association[45] has a good BCS guide, and there are others available online with diagrams from different angles[46,47] and specifically for potbellied pigs.[48] A 1 to 5 scale is used, with 3 representing an ideal body condition and 5 representing an obese animal. Body condition score while the pig is standing.

Tactile assessment of the pig's prominent bony structures, the hips, shoulders, and spine, should also be performed. Feel along the pig's back and assess how easy it is to notice its shoulder blades, hip points, and spine. It should be easy to feel each rib and the hips underneath the skin, but the spine should be padded and not easily felt. If it is not easy to find those points, or they cannot be felt at all, that is a clear sign that the pig is overweight.

Weight loss strategies

Nutritional

Decreasing calorie intake is necessary for weight loss because overweight mini pigs typically expend very few calories through activity due to their environment and mobility. As mentioned above, adult pigs should consume 1% - 2% of their body weight in food based on their ideal body weight. If the overweight pig consumes more than 1% of their body weight, gradually work it lower on this range. Reduce the total amount of food by 5% to 10% per week until the pig starts to lose weight, then stay at that level and re-evaluate after a couple of weeks. Before, during, and after starting a weight loss plan are great times to body condition score pigs. Taking pictures from the same angles and in similar lighting helps monitor progress.

Decrease feed intake gradually and replace high-calorie foods with less calorically-dense foods (ie, higher fiber, lower sugar and protein). Any food outside of the pellets, leafy greens, non-starchy vegetables, and hay should be removed or minimized. Pelleted feed typically constitutes the majority of calories consumed by pet pigs, with the exception of when an inappropriate amount of treats or junk food is fed. Gradually replacing some of the pelleted fed with grass hay and leafy greens dilutes the caloric density of their total diet and increases fiber consumption to help improve satiety. For owners who have poor compliance with a weight loss plan, a recommendation is to set aside the entire day's ration of pellets, produce, and treats in a closed, secure container. As the day progresses, family members may use only this food to feed, train, reward, or enrich their pig.

Behavioral/Environmental

Increasing physical activity is also a critical part of the weight loss equation. Pigs are geared for grazing, rooting, and roaming throughout the day,[3] and these innate behaviors should be incorporated into the feeding plan. Increase the time it takes the pig to eat by scattering their meals to encourage foraging behavior and slow down intake. Food can also be fed in rooting or foraging boxes, treat balls, or puzzle feeders. Hang bags or boxes that contain food and secure it in some way that makes the pig have to work to get it.

Not all enrichment and activity have to be food related. Ideas for non-food related enrichment and activity include toys to push around, manipulate, or chew on, daily walks, newspaper or an old phone book to rip up, and scratch pads. Allowing pigs sufficient outdoor access and time to roam freely is correlated with healthier body condition scores (Shepherd, Wenzel, and Clark, publication in preparation). Lastly, social dynamics must be considered. Dominant pigs in a group eat the most, so ensure sufficient feeding stations are provided to prevent competition. If necessary, monitor pigs while eating to ensure they are not stealing other pigs' portions.

OTHER COMMON NUTRITION CONCERNS OF PET PIG OWNERS
Hoof Health, Arthritis, and Degenerative Joint Disease

Regular hoof trims and maintaining a healthy weight are essential for the pig's life-long mobility and to prevent issues with arthritis, especially in older pigs. Feeding an appropriately balanced diet specific to a mini pig's life stage and providing calcium and phosphorus in the correct ratios and sufficient vitamin D supports proper growth rates and healthy joint development in young pigs.[5] An imbalance in minerals such as zinc, copper, selenium, and manganese or deficiencies in vitamins A, D, and biotin can develop a delicate hoof that is more susceptible to cracks and infections.[49,50]

Dry Skin

Pigs are prone to dry, flaky skin with minimal to severe pruritus.[1] Dry skin is a complex issue affected by many factors, such as genetics, environment, hydration, sun exposure, parasites, bathing, nutrition, and certain health conditions. Nutrients such as vitamins A, E, biotin, and niacin, as well as unsaturated fatty acids, are crucial for maintaining healthy skin because they support skin structure, function, and overall health.

Based on what we know from research in other species and basic nutrient requirements determined for pigs, appropriately balanced mini pig pelleted feeds should be sufficiently fortified in nutrients to prevent skin issues due to nutritional deficiencies. However, if too many other food items are fed that dilute or unbalance the pig's overall nutrition, there may be a nutritional etiology. Fatty acid supplementation can be a long-term remedy; however, caution must be exercised not to promote obesity.

In the absence of a nutritional concern, weather and dehydration are often a culprit in dry skin issues. For most indoor pigs, gently wiping them down with a damp cloth once a week can help remove dry, flaky skin and keep them clean while avoiding over-bathing. Moisturizing lotions or topical coconut oil application can also temporarily alleviate this problem.

SUMMARY

Mini pigs are engaging, intelligent, and entertaining pets that require different management practices compared to other pet species. Pigs need to root, forage, and explore their environment, and this behavior must be a primary consideration when caring for mini pigs. Published nutrient requirements for production pigs are a good reference, but they must be critically interpreted for mini-pig management goals to prioritize longevity and healthy weight maintenance. A balanced diet is based on a pelleted feed formulated for the mini pig's specific life stages and includes vegetables and roughage, with minimal fruit or treats. Mini pigs easily gain weight, and a balanced, high-fiber diet helps maintain healthy body condition to promote longevity and a high quality of life, and reduce the risk of metabolic and joint diseases.

CLINICS CARE POINTS

- A comprehensive diet review, including enrichment and training food items and supplements, is necessary to accurately determine a pig's nutritional balance.
- Body condition scoring is an important tool for appropriate weight management.
- Caloric reduction (through reduced feed intake and caloric density), increased activity, and strict adherence to a long-term weight loss plan are critical to managing obesity in mini pigs.
- Fiber is important for mini pig health, and weight maintenance is often overlooked but can be a valuable tool for nutrition and behavior management.

DISCLOSURE

Dr N.F. Huntley is a nutritionist with Mazuri Exotic Animal Nutrition which markets mini pig diets.

REFERENCES

1. Mozzachio K. Potbellied pig veterinary medicine. St. Louis, MO: Elsevier; 2023.
2. Graves H. Behaviour and ecology of wild and feral swine (Sus scrofa). J Anim Sci 1984;58(2):482–92.
3. Stolba A, Wood-Gush DGM. The behaviour of pigs in a semi-natural environment. Anim Prod 1989;48(2):419–25.
4. Stevens CE, Hume ID. Comparative physiology of the vertebrate digestive system. 2nd edition. New York, NY: Cambridge University Press; 1995.
5. National Research Council (NRC). Nutrient requirements of swine. 11th Revis. Washington, DC: National Academies Press; 2012.
6. Jo H, Kim B. A high correlation between conventional and mini pigs in feed energy utilization. J Anim Sci 2018;96(Suppl. 3):75.
7. Bollen PJA, Madsen LW, Meyer O, et al. Growth differences of male and female Gottingen minipigs during ad libitum feeding: a pilot study. Lab Anim 2005;39(1):80–93.

8. Bollen PJA, Lemmens AG, Beynen AC, et al. Bone composition in male and female Gottingen minipigs fed variously restrictedly and near ad libitum. Scand J Lab Anim Sci 2006;33(3):149–58.

9. Ritskes-Hoitinga J, Bollen PJA. Nutrition of (Gottingen) minipigs: Facts, assumptions and mysteries. Pharmacol Toxicol 1997;80(Suppl. 2):5–9.

10. Liu Y. Fatty acids, inflammation and intestinal health in pigs. J Anim Sci Biotechnol 2015;6(1):1–9.

11. Wallace TC. Health Effects of Coconut Oil—A Narrative Review of Current Evidence. J Am Coll Nutr 2019;38(2):97–107.

12. Agyekum AK, Nyachoti CM. Nutritional and Metabolic Consequences of Feeding High-Fiber Diets to Swine: A Review. Engineering 2017;3(5):716–25.

13. van Milgen J, Noblet J, Dubois S. Energetic Efficiency of Starch, Protein and Lipid Utilization in Growing Pigs. J Nutr 2001;131(4):1309–18.

14. Zhang W, Li D, Liu L, et al. The effects of dietary fiber level on nutrient digestibility in growing pigs. J Anim Sci Biotechnol 2013;4(1):17.

15. Sapkota A, Marchant-Forde JN, Richert BT, et al. Including dietary fiber and resistant starch to increase satiety and reduce aggression in gestating sows1,2. J Anim Sci 2016;94(5):2117–27.

16. Jørgensen H, Theil PK, Bach Knudsen KE. Satiating properties of diets rich in dietary fibre fed to sows as evaluated by physico-chemical properties, gastric emptying rate and physical activity. Livest Sci 2010;134(1–3):37–40.

17. Sánchez D, Miguel M, Aleixandre A. Dietary Fiber, Gut Peptides, and Adipocytokines. J Med Food 2012;15(3):223–30.

18. de Leeuw JA, Bolhuis JE, Bosch G, et al. Effects of dietary fibre on behaviour and satiety in pigs. Proc Nutr Soc 2008;67(4):334–42.

19. Meunier-Salaün MC, Edwards SA, Robert S. Effect of dietary fibre on the behaviour and health of the restricted fed sow. Anim Feed Sci Technol 2001;90(1–2): 53–69.

20. Robert S, Bergeron R, Farmer C, et al. Does the number of daily meals affect feeding motivation and behaviour of gilts fed high-fibre diets? Appl Anim Behav Sci 2002;76(2):105–17.

21. Grześkowiak Ł, Saliu EM, Martínez-Vallespín B, et al. Dietary fiber and its role in performance, welfare, and health of pigs. Anim Health Res Rev 2022;23(2): 165–93.

22. Lindberg JE. Fiber effects in nutrition and gut health in pigs. J Anim Sci Biotechnol 2014;5(1):15.

23. Slavin J. Fiber and Prebiotics: Mechanisms and Health Benefits. Nutrients 2013; 5(4):1417–35.

24. Le Goff G, Noblet J. Comparative total tract digestibility of dietary energy and nutrients in growing pigs and adult sows. J Anim Sci 2001;79(9):2418.

25. Hu R, Li S, Diao H, et al. The interaction between dietary fiber and gut microbiota, and its effect on pig intestinal health. Front Immunol 2023;14:1095740.

26. Koh A, De Vadder F, Kovatcheva-Datchary P, et al. From Dietary Fiber to Host Physiology: Short-Chain Fatty Acids as Key Bacterial Metabolites. Cell 2016; 165(6):1332–45.

27. Li Y, Zhang L, Liu H, et al. Effects of the Ratio of Insoluble Fiber to Soluble Fiber in Gestation Diets on Sow Performance and Offspring Intestinal Development. Animals (Basel) 2019;9(7):422. https://doi.org/10.3390/ani9070422.

28. Jha R, Fouhse JM, Tiwari UP, et al. Dietary Fiber and Intestinal Health of Monogastric Animals. Front Vet Sci 2019;6:48.

29. Owusu-Asiedu A, Patience JF, Laarveld B, et al. Effects of guar gum and cellulose on digesta passage rate, ileal microbial populations, energy and protein digestibility, and performance of grower pigs. J Anim Sci 2006;84(4):843–52.

30. Molist F, de Segura AG, Gasa J, et al. Effects of the insoluble and soluble dietary fibre on the physicochemical properties of digesta and the microbial activity in early weaned piglets. Anim Feed Sci Technol 2009;149(3–4):346–53.

31. Institute of Medicine (US) Panel on the Definition of Dietary Fiber and the Standing Committee on the Scientific Evaluation of Dietary Reference Intakes. Dietary Reference Intakes Proposed Definition of Dietary Fiber. Washington (DC): National Academies Press (US); 2001. Appendix C, Development and Evolution of Methods Used to Extract and Measure Dietary Fiber. Available at: https://www.ncbi.nlm.nih.gov/books/NBK223584/.

32. Baer CK, Ullrey DE, Schlegel ML, et al. Contemporary topics in the nutrition of wild mammals. In: Kleiman DG, Thompson KV, Baer CK, editors. Wild mammals in captivity. 2nd edition. Chicago, IL: University of Chicago Press; 2005. p. 85–103.

33. Schmidt DA, Kerley MS, Porter JH, et al. Structural and nonstructural carbohydrate, fat, and protein composition of commercially available, whole produce. Zoo Biol 2005;24(4):359–73.

34. Stockman J, Fascetti AJ, Kass PH, et al. Evaluation of recipes of home-prepared maintenance diets for dogs. J Am Vet Med Assoc 2013;242(11):1500–5.

35. Oliveira MCC, Brunetto MA, da Silva FL, et al. Evaluation of the owner's perception in the use of homemade diets for the nutritional management of dogs. J Nutr Sci 2014;3:e23.

36. Pedrinelli V, Zafalon RVA, Rodrigues RBA, et al. Influence of number of ingredients, use of supplement and vegetarian or vegan preparation on the composition of homemade diets for dogs and cats. BMC Vet Res 2021;17(1):358.

37. Morris CL. 128 Homemade Pet Diets—What Are the Key Supplement Considerations? J Anim Sci 2021;99(Supplement_3):65–6. https://doi.org/10.1093/jas/skab235.118.

38. Edwards SA. Intake of nutrients from pasture by pigs. Proc Nutr Soc 2003;62(2):257–65.

39. Kim SW, Weaver AC, Shen Y Bin, et al. Improving efficiency of sow productivity: nutrition and health. J Anim Sci Biotechnol 2013;4(1):26.

40. Feyera T, Theil PK. Energy and lysine requirements and balances of sows during transition and lactation: A factorial approach. Livest Sci 2017;201:50–7.

41. Zoran DL. Obesity in Dogs and Cats: A Metabolic and Endocrine Disorder. Vet Clin Small Anim Pract 2010;40(2):221–39.

42. Marshall WG, Bockstahler BA, Hulse DA, et al. A review of osteoarthritis and obesity: current understanding of the relationship and benefit of obesity treatment and prevention in the dog. Vet Comp Orthop Traumatol 2009;22(05):339–45.

43. Salt C, Morris PJ, Wilson D, et al. Association between life span and body condition in neutered client-owned dogs. J Vet Intern Med 2018;33(1):89–99.

44. German AJ, Holden SL, Wiseman-Orr ML, et al. Quality of life is reduced in obese dogs but improves after successful weight loss. Vet J 2012;192(3):428–34.

45. Zolicani C. American Mini Pig Association - What To Do For An Overweight Mini Pig. Published 2015. Accessed May 31, 2023. https://americanminipig association.com/overweight-mini-pig/.

46. The Mini Pig Farrier. Mini Pig Body Condition Scoring and Hoof Health. Published 2022. Accessed May 31, 2023. https://theminipigfarrier.com/mini-pig-body-condition-scoring.

47. Info MP. What does a healthy versus unhealthy pig look like? Published 2020. Accessed May 31, 2023. https://www.minipiginfo.com/mini-pig-body-scoring.html.
48. Virginia Alliance for Potbellied Pigs. Potbellied Pig Body Score.; 2007. Available at: https://nagonline.net/wp-content/uploads/2016/08/Pig-BCS.doc. Accessed May 31, 2023.
49. Misir R, Blair R. Effect of biotin supplementation of a barley-wheat diet on restoration of healthy feet, legs and skin of biotin deficient sows. Res Vet Sci 1986; 40(2):212–8.
50. Langova L, Novotna I, Nemcova P, et al. Impact of Nutrients on the Hoof Health in Cattle. Animals 2020;10(10):1824.

Assisted Enteral Feeding of Exotic Companion Animals

Y. Becca Leung, BSc, BVSc, PhD, Dipl. ACVIM (Nutrition)

KEYWORDS

• Nutrition • Hospital • Exotic • Pet • Rabbit • Ferret • Reptile • Avian

KEY POINTS

- The prevalence and negative consequences of malnutrition in hospitalized exotic companion animal species are unknown but they have been established in human medicine and veterinary medicine for dogs and cats.
- Monitoring the nutritional status of patients should be done frequently with the use of calibrated scales for body weight and body condition scoring.
- Energy equations provide an estimation of requirements, and so should be adapted to fit the individual and their nutritional goals during hospitalization.
- Nutritional support should be provided in a timely manner for patients with high metabolic rates, which is relevant for many exotic companion animals.

INTRODUCTION

The world of exotic companion animals is great and ever expanding. It includes a large variety of families, genera, and species, all of which have very different dietary requirements and nutritional needs. As such, it can be difficult to discuss each species in detail within a single article. Therefore, this article will focus on general nutritional considerations during the hospitalization of exotic patients, with specific references to species when appropriate.

In 2011, the World Small Animal Veterinary Association (WSAVA) added "nutritional assessment" as the 5th Vital Assessment which should be performed in all patients, following temperature, pulse, respiration, and pain assessment.[1] Although this recommendation is focused on small animals, particularly dogs and cats, there should be an equal recognition of the importance of nutrition in our exotic companion animal patients. A challenge for veterinarians lies in understanding how to recognize malnutrition in various species and how to address it. Although there is active research in this topic and a growing understanding as to the specific needs of individual species, much more work is needed, particularly in understanding how to provide the best nutritional support during convalescence.

Veterinary Nutrition Group, Sydney, Australia
E-mail address: dr.becca.leung@gmail.com

Vet Clin Exot Anim 27 (2024) 115–134
https://doi.org/10.1016/j.cvex.2023.08.003
1094-9194/24/© 2023 Elsevier Inc. All rights reserved.

MALNUTRITION

Malnourishment is a nutritional state that results from a lack of intake or uptake of nutrients, leading to an altered body composition, reduced physical and mental function, and impaired clinical outcomes.[2] The term malnutrition can be used to describe both under- and overnutrition. In the case of hospitalized patients, however, evidence from humans, dogs, and cats indicates that undernutrition in the form of hyporexia and anorexia is most common; a substantial portion of patients entering the hospital arrive in a malnourished state or subsequently become undernourished during hospitalization.[3–6] Little, if any, is known about the prevalence of malnutrition in hospitalized, exotic companion animal species. However, it is hypothesized by this author to be similar.

The mechanism behind a reduction in food intake during periods of illness, particularly with concurrent pyrexia, is an evolutionarily conserved trait that is apparent throughout the animal kingdom. It is believed to be an acute phase response to the release of cytokines IL-1β and TNF-α, which act on the hypothalamus and reduces appetite.[7–9] Increasing the nutritional status of hospitalized humans, dogs, and cats has been shown to improve outcomes including reduced postoperative infections, shorter hospitalization, and a reduced risk of mortality.[10–12] In dogs and cats, malnutrition in the hospital occurs due to food refusal, nausea, and poorly written dietary instructions by caretakers.[6,13] In a study of hospitalized dogs, 16% lost weight during hospitalization and the majority (84%) of the dogs consumed less than 25% of their resting energy requirement (RER) on average.[6]

Nutritional Assessments

As the consequences of malnutrition is likely relevant during the hospitalization of exotic species as well, clinicians should be able to determine which patients are at risk of malnutrition, assess their nutritional status, and intervene when necessary. The WSAVA Nutritional Assessment Guidelines nutritional screening risk factors can be adapted for use in exotic companion animal patients.[1] Risk factors include a history of gastrointestinal dysfunction and being fed diets that are not suitable for the species. A particular challenge for exotic patients is that some species naturally undergo periods of fasting. Therefore, special consideration should be made to the natural cycle of inactivity and reduced intake during brumation in certain reptiles and amphibians, and torpor in birds.

There are several methods to assess malnutrition, with body weight (BW) and body condition scoring (BCS) as the most widely used in dogs and cats in clinical practice.[14] Daily (or as often as practical) monitoring of BW using the same, calibrated scale should be done in all patients. This will allow for the rapid detection of BW changes. However, changes in BW are not necessarily indicative of body composition (ie, fat and lean mass) changes. One use of a BCS system is to be able to estimate the percentage of body fat mass and to use this, along with current BW, to estimate lean mass and ideal BW. The BCS system has been validated for dogs and cats and every change in BCS score in a 1 to 9 scale equates to approximately a 5% change in body fat mass.[15,16] There are BCS scales available for several species including rabbits, guinea pigs, ferrets, birds, snakes, frogs, lizards, and turtles.[17–28] They have various levels of validation, however, so caution should be taken if using to estimate fat mass % and ideal weight.

In addition, BCS can be helpful as a tool to monitor the nutrition status of a given patient, even after being discharged from the hospital. In one study, researchers found that a rabbit body scoring system had good repeatability between veterinarians and owners.[18] Body fat is a good energy reserve, and useful as a marker of nutritional status. For small mammals such as rabbits and guinea pigs, the areas of the body for palpation are similar to those of dogs and cats. However, a challenge remains in understanding the right location to examine body fat mass for other species as these may be different. In birds, subcutaneous fat deposits can be appreciated as a visual representation of energy storage, although the site varies by species.[29] Further, the use of morphometric measurements is commonplace for exotic species. Like the body mass index used in humans, ratios are derived using the BW of an animal divided by some measure of size. A novel measurement in rabbits (a ratio of BW to dorsal fore-limb length) was found to be useful in 'medium-sized' rabbits to estimate body fat mass.[27] In lizards, a measurement of BW over snout-vent length was found to be moderately correlated to body fat mass as measured by dual-energy X-ray absorptiometry.[30]

When caloric intake is insufficient for a prolonged period, or if there is protein-energy malnutrition, amino acids can be used for energy through the gluconeogenesis pathway. However, it is not beneficial to lose muscle simply for amino acid provision and energy generation. In addition, an increase in protein catabolism (termed cachexia) can occur in hospital patients as the result of the underlying disease(s), which is not reversible using conventional nutritional interventions.[31,32] Preservation of lean mass is thought to be important in hospitalized patients. Having low muscle mass at admission and/or losing muscle during hospitalization are associated with negative prognoses and outcomes in human patients.[33]

A muscle condition scoring (MCS) system has been developed for dogs and cats. However, MCS has been shown to only be weekly correlated with total lean mass in dogs.[34] A better correlation between MCS and lean mass has been demonstrated in cats.[35] In avians, palpation of the pectoral muscle mass and assessment of the prominence of the keel is a method of assessing muscle mass (**Fig. 1**). However, considerations of the patient's lifestyle and home environment should be made as activity can also affect overall muscling. While muscle loss is a marker of malnutrition, it also can influence outcome by affecting the mobility and strength of a patient.[36]

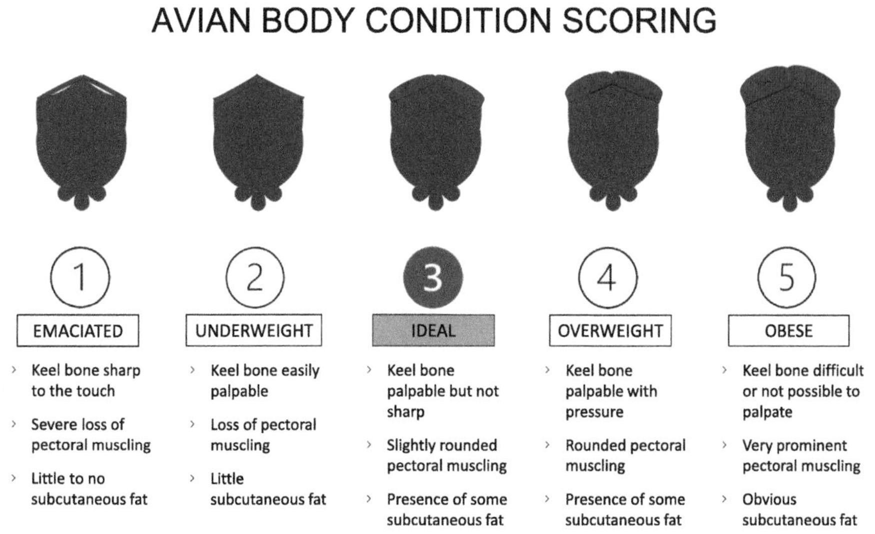

AVIAN BODY CONDITION SCORING

① EMACIATED	② UNDERWEIGHT	③ IDEAL	④ OVERWEIGHT	⑤ OBESE
› Keel bone sharp to the touch	› Keel bone easily palpable	› Keel bone palpable but not sharp	› Keel bone palpable with pressure	› Keel bone difficult or not possible to palpate
› Severe loss of pectoral muscling	› Loss of pectoral muscling	› Slightly rounded pectoral muscling	› Rounded pectoral muscling	› Very prominent pectoral muscling
› Little to no subcutaneous fat	› Little subcutaneous fat	› Presence of some subcutaneous fat	› Presence of some subcutaneous fat	› Obvious subcutaneous fat

Fig. 1. Body condition scoring tool for avian species.

As no method is sufficient on its own, it is recommended to use BW and body condition (fat and lean mass) to assess and monitor the nutritional status of patients. These measures should be done consistently and frequently.

FEEDING IN HOSPITAL

To better understand the nutritional needs of exotic companion animal patients, it is first helpful to understand some general nutrition concepts, namely the function of macronutrients (fat, protein, carbohydrates) and micronutrients (vitamins and minerals), particularly during disease and illness. Exotic companion animals have wide-ranging nutritional needs, and often, specific requirements have not been defined. For some small mammals and avian species, energy and nutrient requirements have been established for laboratory or agricultural production use, and not for health and longevity. In addition, little is understood about specific needs during hospitalization and recovery. Although we can speak about key concepts and generalities, we should take care to ensure that nutritional considerations should be made with each species' particularities in mind.

Energy

The main goal for any hospitalized patient is to ensure they consume sufficient, but not excessive, amounts of food to meet their energy requirements. Although a simple task in theory, practically, it can be more difficult which is highlighted by how common weight loss is in hospitalized patients. Studies of dogs demonstrated that 15% to 45% of patients lost weight during their hospitalization.[5,6] The basal metabolic rate makes up the majority of an animal's total energy expenditure, and describes an individual's metabolism in an awake, fasted, and resting state in a thermoneutral environment.[37] This most commonly describes the situation for hospitalized patients and is defined as the RER of a patient. However, maintenance energy requirements (MER) are also often calculated for hospitalized exotic companion animal species.[38,39]

A hypermetabolic state can occur with acute injury or infections. This leads to insulin and growth hormone resistance, and results in the catabolism of endogenous stores of protein, fats, and carbohydrates.[40] However, the challenge is that the metabolic response to injury, surgery, inflammation, and stress cannot be accurately predicted and evolves over the course of illness, so the risk of over or under estimating requirement in this state can be significant.[41] In critically ill human patients undergoing mechanical ventilation, less than half were considered hypermetabolic and the majority were overfed, receiving greater than 110% of their required calories as measured using indirect calorimetry.[42] Because of this and the consequences of overfeeding (which will be explored shortly), the use of an illness factor to increase energy provision not favored anymore.

Energy equations for hospitalized exotic companion animal patients can be found in **Table 1**. It is important to remember that these equations are for estimating a patient's requirement and adjustments are likely needed. BW is commonly used to estimate energy requirements; however, considerations should be made on the tissue composition of the patient. Lean tissues, and in particular lean organ tissue, have a much greater metabolic rate compared with fatty tissues.[43,44] Although an overweight animal has a greater mass of both lean and fat compared with an ideally conditioned animal, the majority is an excess of fat.[15,16] As such, using current BW in individuals with obesity may lead to an overestimation of energy requirements. In humans, total energy expenditure does not increase linearly with increasing weight and instead scales with lean mass.[45] In addition, in cats, lean mass has been shown to be a better

Table 1
Starting energy equations for adult exotic companion animal species

Species	Energy	Equation (kcals/day)	Reference
Rat	MER[a]	110 x body weight (kg) $^{0.75}$	Bullen,[137] 2021
Mice	MER	110 x body weight (kg) $^{0.75}$	Bullen,[137] 2021
Rabbit	MER	100 x body weight (kg) $^{0.75}$	Bullen,[137] 2021
Guinea pig	MER	110 x body weight (kg) $^{0.75}$	Bullen,[137] 2021
Ferret	MER	200–300 x body weight (kg) $^{0.75}$	Johnson-Delaney,[138] 2014
Passerines	BMR[b]	129 x body weight (kg) $^{0.75}$	Beaufrère,[39] 2021
Nonpasserines	BMR	78 x body weight (kg) $^{0.75}$	Beaufrère,[39] 2021
Reptiles[c]	BMR	32 x body weight (kg) $^{0.75}$	Donoghue & McKeown,[139] 1999

[a] Maintenance energy requirement (MER).
[b] Basal metabolic rate (BMR).
[c] Environmental temperature of 30°C/86°F.

predictor of MER compared with BW.[46] However, as hospital patients are at risk of malnutrition and often lose weight, it is of this author's opinion that current BW should be used when estimating the energy requirements of hospitalized patients. However, BW should be monitored daily, and intake adjusted accordingly to meet nutritional goals. In underweight patients, using current BW to calculate requirements is indicated, particularly in emaciated patients (BCS 1–2 out of 9), to reduce the risk of refeeding syndrome.

Refeeding Syndrome

Refeeding syndrome occurs during the reintroduction of food after a period of prolonged starvation. The sudden rise in blood glucose leads to a release of insulin and the uptake of phosphorus, magnesium, potassium, and thiamin intracellularly. The rapid decline in these nutrient concentrations in circulation leads to complications including hemolytic anemia, muscle weakness, ataxia, cardiac and respiratory abnormalities, and neurologic dysfunction.[47] The syndrome has been described in several species, including small ruminants, donkeys, cats, dogs, and chickens, and is believed to be possible in other species as well.[48–52]

To reduce the risk of a patient developing refeeding syndrome, it is advised to feed at-risk patients a diet containing low to moderate amounts of digestible carbohydrates and to reintroduce food slowly. In addition, it is important to monitor serum phosphate, magnesium, and potassium before and after feeding. Thiamin is not easily monitored in patients, and so presuming sufficient intake of this nutrient requires provision of an appropriate diet and/or supplementation, in addition to careful monitoring of clinical signs. **Box 1** contains examples of factors that increase the risk of developing refeeding syndrome in humans.[53] To avoid this, feeding amounts should start as a percentage of a patient's RER (typically 25%–33%) and increased daily as tolerated until their full RER is reached.

Fat and Essential Fatty Acids

Dietary fat is an integral energy source for the body in addition to a source of essential fatty acids, fat-soluble vitamins A, D, E, and K, phospholipids, sphingolipids, steroids, and eicosanoids. The main metabolic product of fatty acid oxidation is acetyl-CoA, which can enter the tricarboxylic acid cycle or be used to synthesize other lipids.

> **Box 1**
> **Factors that increase the risk of refeeding syndrome in human patients which are relevant to exotic companion animal patients[53]**
>
> Postoperative patients
>
> Elderly patients (comorbidities, decreased physiologic reserve)
>
> Patients with uncontrolled diabetes mellitus (electrolyte depletion, diuresis)
>
> Patients with chronic malnutrition (marasmus, kwashiorkor, prolong fasting or low energy diet, morbid obesity, high stress in patients unfed for > 7 days, malabsorptive syndrome)
>
> Long term users of antacids (magnesium and aluminum salts)
>
> Long term users of diuretics (loss of electrolytes)
>
> Oncology patients

Ketones are fat metabolites that play a vital role in survival during long-term fasting or starvation by sparing glucose and limiting the need for gluconeogenesis. Ketogenesis occurs mainly in hepatocytes and intestinal epithelial cells, but is also reported to occur in other tissues at lower rates.[54,55] The concentration of ketones present in circulation during fasting varies between species; humans have a more rapid rise compared with rodents, rabbits, guinea pigs, and dogs when fasted for a similar amount of time.[56,57] In avians, the use of blood ketones has been proposed to correlate with the length of fasting.[58] In reptiles, some species have an increase in circulating ketones during fasting, whereas others have a decrease, which may indicate a reduction in metabolic rate in response to the fast.[59]

Each gram of fat provides over twice the energy compared to either a gram of protein or carbohydrates. A benefit of using more fat in a diet is to decrease the volume needed to be fed to meet energy requirements. This can be helpful when performing assisted feeding. However, excess dietary fat, particularly when there is fat maldigestion and malabsorption, can lead to steatorrhea and negative effects such as increased Toll-like receptor signaling, intestinal permeability, endotoxin translocation, and inflammatory cytokine production.[60,61] Additional considerations where dietary fat may need to be restricted include patients with hyperlipidemia, lymphangiectasia, or chylous effusion.

Linoleic acid and alpha-linolenic acid are polyunsaturated fatty acids that play important roles in ceramide production, immunity, and reproduction. They are established as essential fatty acids in some species, including growing and reproducing dogs, cats, rats, and poultry.[62–64] Longer chain fatty acids, including eicosapentaenoic acid and docosahexaenoic acid, have other biological functions, including the modulation of inflammatory pathways and retinal and brain development.[65–67] Although the essentiality of these fats has not been established in all exotic companion animals, it is precautionarily recommended to include these fats into their diets.

Protein and Essential Amino Acids

The total amount of protein in a diet is important, as are the constituents. Dietary proteins provide a source of essential and nonessential amino acids, which are required for a variety of functions including the synthesis and degradation of tissues, immune function, and hormone production, to name a few. The required amount of protein to feed depends on the species, with obligate carnivores, such as ferrets and snakes, requiring the most. Arginine is an essential amino acid for obligate carnivores as well.

Feeding a single meal containing little or no arginine leads to hyperammonemia and signs of encephalopathy in cats and ferrets within hours.[68,69]

Another consideration in addition to the total amount of protein in a diet is its digestibility. A strategy to increase protein digestibility is through hydrolyzation. The provision of peptides from hydrolyzed proteins has been shown to improve overall digestibility and speed of the absorption compared with intact proteins.[70] However, other studies indicate that the benefits of peptides over intact proteins may be limited.[71] Thus, the advantage of feeding hydrolyzed proteins over highly digestible, intact proteins remains to be determined in hospitalized patients.

In certain disease conditions, the amount of protein fed may need to be restricted. This includes patients with protein-losing nephropathies and hepatic encephalopathies.[72–74] In other cases, supplementation of amino acids may be of beneficial. Glutamine is not an essential amino acid, but may be conditionally essential in times of reproduction and growth in some species, and plasma glutamine has been shown to be low during critical illness in human patients.[75,76] However, there are inconsistent results in studies showing a benefit of supplementing glutamine in critically ill patients in intensive care units (ICU). In human medicine, supplementation in patients with severe burns and complicated wound healing is recommended, but not in patients with liver or renal disease.[77]

Carbohydrates

Carbohydrates can be provided as small units (sugars) or as more complex molecules (starches, glycogen, and fibers). The main function of digestible carbohydrates is to provide a source of energy for organisms. They can be metabolized shortly after ingestion or can be stored as glycogen molecules in the body. Glycogen stores are generally reported to be depleted after 24 hours of fasting, although the previous diet, activity, and species differences can influence this rate.[78,79] The ease to which the body can extract energy from dietary carbohydrates depends on the structure of the molecule and how the carbohydrates are processed. Starches have improved digestibility after cooking and the gelatinization process. Even in obligate carnivores, such as the cat, they able to digest nearly 100% of cooked cornstarch compared with only 60% to 70% of raw cornstarch.[80,81]

Hyperglycemia is a common clinical feature in critically ill patients.[82–84] In veterinary patients receiving parenteral nutrition, hyperglycemia is the most common metabolic complication, followed by hyperlipidemia and hyperbilirubinemia.[85,86] The consequences of being in a hyperglycemia state occurs in cells which are slow to downregulate transport, such as vascular endothelial, mesangial and neuronal cells.[87–89] This causes the glycation of intracellular proteins and reactive oxygen species generation, which can lead to cellular dysfunction, vasculitis, and impaired wound healing. In human patients, preventing hyperglycemia has been shown to reduce complications, the length of hospitalization, and overall mortality.[90,91] In hospitalized dogs and cats, patients commonly presented in a hyperglycemia state or developed hyperglycemia while in the hospital, which was associated with longer hospitalization.[92,93] As such, recommendations in human medicine include limiting the amount of digestible carbohydrates fed and careful monitoring of blood glucose for patients in the ICU.[77]

Although much less is known about hyperglycemic events during hospitalization in exotic companion animal species, avoiding excess digestible carbohydrates seems prudent in those critically ill. It is important however not confuse digestible carbohydrates with nondigestible carbohydrates, which are more commonly known as fibers. The importance of dietary fibers depends on the species; for instance, rabbits and guinea pigs require fibers to maintain gut motility, luminal pH, and a normal microbiota.

The total dietary fiber requirement for rabbits and guinea pigs is greater than or equal to 15% of the diet on a dry matter basis.[94,95] In contrast, some other species have a digestive system more suited to a low fiber diet, such as the ferret. In these species, excessive fiber can lead to a variety of side effects including diarrhea or constipation, bloating, and abdominal pain. In addition, increased fiber can also reduce the overall digestibility of a diet in addition to binding to minerals, reducing their bioavailability.[96,97] As such, the fiber contents of diets fed during hospitalization should be tailored to the species intended.

Micronutrients

Vitamins take part in a wide range of functions including as cofactors for enzymes in metabolic processes. Some vitamins are essential, and a deficiency can develop if they are not consumed in adequate quantities. However, the depletion of vitamins occurs at different rates in the body depending on their storage. Fat-soluble vitamins include vitamin A, D, E, and K, are stored in adipose tissues and liver, and are depleted at a relatively slower rate compared with water-soluble vitamins such as B vitamins and ascorbic acid (vitamin C). However, absorption of fat-soluble vitamins may be compromised when fat maldigestion and malabsorption is present in a patient.[98] In a study of hospitalized dogs, those who were critically ill or those with sepsis were found to have lower serum 25-hydroxycholecalciferol compared with healthy, control dogs.[99]

Guinea pigs are unable to synthesize vitamin C endogenously from glucose due a low activity of L-gluconolactone oxidase enzyme, and so must receive this nutrient from their diet.[100] Vitamin C is needed for the production of hydroxylysine and hydroxyproline, which are building blocks for collagen and important for wound healing.[101,102] It also plays an important role in the endogenous antioxidant pathway. The requirement for vitamin C for guinea pigs is believed to be around 200 mg/kg diet.[62] The requirement for additional vitamin C during hospitalized in guinea pigs is not known. Humans also have an essentiality for vitamin C, and a reduction in circulating vitamin C has been described in critically ill patients despite supplementation.[103,104] Caution should be taken, however, to avoid overzealous supplementation, as all nutrients are toxic at some level (even water). Although vitamin C is generally thought of as having low toxicity, feeding a protein-deficient diet in addition to high doses of vitamin C has been shown to cause toxicity in guinea pigs.[105] In addition, chronic intake of very high doses of vitamin C (8500 mg/kg diet) has been found to be associated with increased TGF-β activation and cartilage damage in guinea pigs.[106]

Minerals take part in a wide variety of bodily functions including structural, maintenance of acid-base and water balance, blood pressure, electrical conduction, and hormone and immune function.[107] Ensuring a diet is replete with essential minerals is important for patients, although the exact amounts required is often unknown. Supplementation is not normally recommended without evidence of a deficiency. In human medicine, supplementation with nutrients that take part in the antioxidant pathway, such as selenium, is not indicated unless there is a deficiency.[77] Some serum metabolites related to mineral status are available commercially and can be used to help with a patient's nutritional assessment. However, care should be taken when interpreting results in relation to provided laboratory reference intervals, as small sample sizes and lack of method standardization can affect their utility.[108,109]

VOLUNTARY CONSUMPTION

Voluntary oral feeding is the ideal goal for all patients. In exotic companion animal species, providing adequate husbandry, including temperature and humidity, is important not only for recovery, but also can increase the likelihood of voluntary food consumption. Other factors that may help include offering the same food as fed at home, limiting handling, covering cage doors with sheets/towels, and minimizing external noises. Diets and water should be provided at room temperature and uneaten food items removed often to reduce contamination and the risk of food aversion. In addition, providing basking lamps and water baths for reptiles and aquatic species may also encourage food consumption.[50]

The use of antiemetics and appetite stimulants has been used successfully in some exotic companion animal species, including rabbits and budgerigars.[110–112] However, species differences in metabolism and biotransformation of drugs, especially during disease states, have not been well established. So, it is important to look for evidence of not only efficacy, but safety in the short and long-term use of appetite stimulants in the particular species of interest.

While voluntary feeding is the goal, often, nutritional support is needed in hospitalized patients. The WSAVA guidelines advise that interventional nutritional support should occur for patients who have not eaten sufficiently for approximately 3 to 5 days, including the days before hospitalization.[1] In humans, critically ill patients in ICU are considered at risk for malnutrition after 48 hours.[77] However, for species with high metabolic rates, which is the case for many exotic companion animal species, the risk of malnutrition and the need for intervention may need to occur sooner. Ensuring adequate hydration should always occur before the nutritional intervention, and the contribution of water in the diet and any used for flushing a feeding tube should be considered when calculating total water intake.

ASSISTED FEEDING

If voluntary intake by a patient is insufficient to meet energy and nutrient requirements, assisted feeding is required. Types of assisted feeding include hand feeding, syringe feeding, gavage feeding, and the use of enteral feeding tubes. The most appropriate option for a patient should depend on several factors, including the patient's nutritional status, functionality of their gastrointestinal tract, their ability to undergo general anesthesia, the intended duration of nutritional support, and diet availability.[113]

Hand feeding and syringe feeding can be short-term solutions to supplement voluntary intake and to stimulate appetite. However, these methods are often not very rewarding as it can be very time consuming, and the volume given is often insufficient to meet total energy requirements. Another challenge of these types of forced feeding is that learned taste aversion can occur when consumption of a food is associated with nausea and/or vomiting, particularly with the introduction of new foods. This has been documented in humans, dogs, cats, and several exotic companion animal species including rabbits, ferrets, blackbirds, and lizards.[114–120] This conserved phenomenon is a learned behavior with evolutionary benefits by teaching an organism to avoid food containing potentially toxic compounds.[121] Therefore, introduction of novel foods intended for long-term feeding during hospitalization is not advised without strict control of nausea and other gastrointestinal signs.

Gavage (orogastric) feeding is similar to syringe feeding, although it can take less time and generally, more volume is able to be administered. Avian species and reptiles are more amendable to this type of feeding, and red rubber tubes or straight/curved ball-tipped metal gavage feeding tubes are often used. The size of the tube depends on the species but can range from small to large (18–8 gauge). Using an oral speculum can help with access to the oral cavity and passage of the feeding tube. Complications can include aspiration (if food is introduced into the respiratory tract) and laceration

Table 2
List of commercially available diets suitable to tube feeding

Species	Manufacturer	Diet name	Min. Tube Size suitability[c]	Energy (kcal/kg dry Weight)	Max. Crude Fiber (% as-fed)	Protein (%ME)	Fat (%ME)	Digestible CHO (% ME)
Rabbit Guinea pigs Reptiles Tortoises	EmerAid[d]	Intensive Care Herbivore	5 Fr	2950	35.7	27.0[c]	33.2[c]	39.6[c]
	EmerAid	Sustain Herbivore	Syringeable	3040	26.0	19.1[b]	29.3[b]	51.6[b]
	Oxbow[e]	Critical Care Herbivore Apple-Banana	Syringeable	2660	26.0	25.6[b]	17.0[b]	57.4[b]
	Oxbow	Critical Care Fine Grind Papaya	5 Fr	2660	26.0	25.6[b]	17.0[b]	57.4[b]
Parrots Doves Chickens Finches Canaries Gamebirds Sugar glider Squirrel Mice and rats Gerbil, hamster, hedgehog, bearded dragon, chameleon, skink, turtle[a]	EmerAid	Intensive Care Omnivore	5 Fr	4086	3.9	22.3[c]	30.1[c]	47.8[c]
	Oxbow	Critical Care Omnivore	Syringeable	3600	3.0	23.3[b]	30.0[b]	46.7[b]

Species	Manufacturer	Diet	Tube size						
Ferret	EmerAid	Intensive Care Carnivore	5 Fr		4979	4.9	29.1[c]	62.1[c]	8.9[c]
Fox									
Birds of prey									
Frogs									
Toads									
Lizards									
Snakes									
	Oxbow	Critical Care Carnivore	Syringeable		6000	3.0	30.0[b]	48.0[b]	22.0[b]
	Royal Canin[f]	Recovery canned	12 Fr		986	3.1	38[c]	58[c]	4[c]
	Royal Canin	Recovery liquid	5 Fr		880	0.1	32[c]	48[c]	20[c]

Abbreviations: CHO, carbohydrates; ME, metabolizable energy.

[a] Appropriate when mixed with either intensive care herbivore or carnivore.
[b] Calculated using At-water factors (4 kcal/g protein, 9 kcal/g fat, 4 kcal/g carbohydrates).
[c] Reported by the manufacturer.
[d] EmerAid, LLC, Cornell, IL, USA
[e] Oxbow Animal Health, Murdock, NE, USA
[f] Royal Canin SAS, Aimargues, France.

of the oropharynx, esophagus, or crop if the tube is introduced too forcefully. The insertion length of the tube for gavage should depend on the location of the crop or stomach of the patient. An estimation of crop volume in birds ranges from 20 to 50 mL/kg BW.[122,123] In critically ill patients, it is advised to start with multiple small meals a day at a percentage of RER, and to increase based on clinical signs and tolerance by the patient.

Placement of enteral feeding tubes can allow for easier feeding with less manipulation, and has been shown to improve clinical outcomes in canine patients with parvoviral enteritis and septic peritonitis.[11,12] The use of feeding tubes to provide enteral nutrition is preferred over parenteral nutrition in order preserve intestinal villous function and motility.[124,125] The use of parenteral nutrition is recommended for those patients who have severe gastrointestinal disfunction or moribund with a risk of aspiration.

Feeding tubes are named based on their anatomic location in the body, and their size described as French units (commonly abbreviated as "Fr"). One French unit is equal to 0.33 mm. To determine the diameter of a feeding tube, divide the French unit by 3. For instance, a 5 Fr feeding tube would have a 1.7 mm outside diameter. This does not describe the luminal diameter, however, and this can differ between manufacturers. The size of the lumen ultimately dictates the type and viscosity of food that can be used. Feeding tubes which enter through the nose include nasoesophageal, nasogastric, and nasojejunal tube. These tubes are limited in size (3.5–8 Fr) and can be made of polyurethane, silicone, and polyvinyl chloride. Polyvinyl chloride (PVC) is less commonly used due to its stiffness, hardening properties, especially when exposed to gastric acids, and low biocompatability.[126–128] For smaller tubes, using less viscous diets and a small syringe for feeding can help reduce pressure and improve flow.

Complications of nasal feeding tubes include epistaxis, nasal discharge, kinking, tube obstruction, and tube displacement, which can lead to aspiration. In addition, nasogastric and nasojejunal tubes traverse the lower esophageal sphincter, which may increase the risk of reflux, particularly with larger-size tubes. In a study of human infants, patients with feeding tubes that entered the stomach had to more episodes of reflux compared with those where the tubes which remained in their esophagus.[129] In another study, adult patients with percutaneous endoscopic gastrostomy tubes had less occurrence of esophagitis compared with those with nasogastric tubes.[130] However, in a study of hospitalized dogs, there was no difference in complications between those with nasoesophageal compared with nasogastric feeding tubes.[131]

Esophagostomy tubes are commonly used as medium and long-term feeding devices in exotic companion animal species. They require anesthesia for placement, but as they are larger (8–14 Fr), they allow for more flexibility in feeding. These tubes are generally better tolerated than nasoenteral tubes and can be sent home for long-term use by clients. In cats with chronic kidney disease, esophagostomy tubes have been used to maintain, or even improve body condition score, over several months.[132] Complications include dermatitis, infection, and leakage around the stoma site. Esophagostomy tubes are available in several materials similarly to nasoenteral tubes, with the addition of red rubber. The use of red rubber tubes can be desirable as they are relatively inexpensive, but they harden and cause a local reaction similarly to PVC. The length of the esophagostomy tube typically extends until the distal third of esophagus in mammals, but can extend into the stomach in birds and reptiles.[113]

Gastrostomy feeding tubes are indicated for long-term nutritional support. These tubes are typically made of latex or silicone, which have limited stiffening and have the largest diameter (up to 30 Fr typically). Complications include erythema, cellulitis, infection, and leaking around the stoma site as well as tube kinking, displacement, and premature removal, which could lead to peritonitis if food particles leak into the peritoneum.[133] Marking the end of the tube as it exits the skin can help with monitoring for displacement. In addition, careful placement and tube management can limit these complications. Other feeding tube types such as duodenostomy and jejunosotmy tubes are also possible, but are not commonly used.[113]

Before feeding, verification of the tube location is vital. The gold standard for assessing placement is to use imaging.[128,134] Other methods include aspirating to determine negative pressure or stomach contents or instilling water or air and/or attaching a capnograph, both of which are fallible. The use of a capnograph seems to be a more accurate method to confirm location, although this has not been evaluated in exotic companion animals.[135,136] A list of commercially available diets that could be used for tube feeding are provided in **Table 2**. A final important consideration is the positioning of animal during and after feeding. The goal is to position the patient in a natural, relaxed state that encourages normal gastrointestinal motility and movement of food into the distal parts of the gastrointestinal tract. After feeding, placing patients back into their cage and minimizing stressors including noise may help with reducing the risk of regurgitation. Finally, removal of the feeding tube should not occur until the patient begins to voluntarily eat sufficiently for several days in a row.

SUMMARY

The importance of preventing and alleviating malnutrition is clear in hospitalized human, dogs, and cats. Although there is a need for further evidence of a similar benefit in exotic companion animal patients, there are enough similarities in metabolism and function that it can be hypothesized to be the same. As such, a nutritional assessment is recommended to be performed routinely on all patients and assisted feeding implemented when needed.

CLINICS CARE POINTS

- Malnutrition is commonly documented in hospitalized humans, canine and feline patients, and is associated with negative consequences. Although less is known about exotic companion animal species, there are likely similarities.

- Energy and nutrient requirements have not been defined for many exotic companion animal species. In addition, even for those which have requirements established, they are based on production factors, rather than for health and longevity.

- Monitoring the nutritional status of patients should be done frequently using body weight and measures of lean and fat mass. Nutritional interventions likely need to occur earlier in some exotic species with a higher metabolic rate compared with humans, dogs, and cats.

DISCLOSURE

The author declares no conflicts of interest with respect to the research, authorship, or publication of this article.

REFERENCES

1. Freeman L, Becvarova I, Cave N, et al. WSAVA nutritional assessment guidelines. J Small Anim Pract 2011;52(7):385–96.
2. Cederholm T, Barazzoni R, Austin P, et al. ESPEN guidelines on definitions and terminology of clinical nutrition. Clin Nutr 2017;36(1):49–64.

3. Correia MITD, Perman MI, Waitzberg DL. Hospital malnutrition in Latin America: A systematic review. Clin Nutr 2017;36(4):958–67.

4. Chandler ML, Gunn-moore DA. Nutritional status of canine and feline patients admitted to a referral veterinary internal medicine service. J Nutr 2004;134(8): 2050S–2S.

5. Brunetto Ma, Gomes MOSS, Andre MR, et al. Effects of nutritional support on hospital outcome in dogs and cats. J Vet Emerg Crit Care 2010;20(2):224–31.

6. Molina J, Hervera M, Manzanilla EG, et al. Evaluation of the prevalence and risk factors for undernutrition in hospitalized dogs. Front Vet Sci 2018;5(AUG):1–8.

7. Hart BL. The behavior of sick animals. Vet Clin North Am Small Anim Pract 1991; 21(2):225–37.

8. Adamo SA, Bartlett A, Le J, et al. Illness-induced anorexia may reduce trade-offs between digestion and immune function. Anim Behav 2010;79(1):3–10.

9. Asarian L, Langhans W. A new look on brain mechanisms of acute illness anorexia. Physiol Behav 2010;100(5):464–71.

10. Haac B, Henry S, Diaz J, et al. Early enteral nutrition is associated with reduced morbidity in critically ill soft tissue patients. Am Surg 2018;84(6):1003–9.

11. Liu DT, Brown DC, Silverstein DC. Early nutritional support is associated with decreased length of hospitalization in dogs with septic peritonitis: A retrospective study of 45 cases (2000–2009). J Vet Emerg Crit Care 2012;22(4):453–9.

12. Mohr AJ, Leisewitz AL, Jacobson LS, et al. Effect of early enteral nutrition on intestinal permeability, intestinal protein loss, and outcome in dogs with severe parvoviral enteritis. J Vet Intern Med 2003;17(6):791–8.

13. Remillard RL, Darden DE, Michel KE, et al. An investigation of the relationship between caloric intake and outcome in hospitalized dogs. Vet Ther 2001;2(4): 301–10. Available at: http://www.ncbi.nlm.nih.gov/pubmed/19746652.

14. Santarossa A, Parr JM, Verbrugghe A. Assessment of canine and feline body composition by veterinary health care teams in Ontario, Canada. Can Vet J 2018;59(12):1280–6.

15. Laflamme D. Development and validation of a body condition score system for dogs. Canine Pract 1997;22(4):10–5.

16. Laflamme D. Development and validation of a body condition score system for cats: a clinical tool. Feline Pract 1997;25:13–8.

17. Schulte-Hostedde AI, Millar JS, Hickling GJ. Evaluating body condition in small mammals. Can J Zool 2001;79(6):1021–9.

18. Thompson JL, Koh P, Meredith AL, et al. Preliminary investigations into the use of the five-point body condition scale (Size-O-Meter) and its use in pet owner education. J Exot Pet Med 2019;31:95–9.

19. Warner DA, Johnson MS, Nagy TR. Validation of Body Condition Indices and Quantitative Magnetic Resonance in Estimating Body Composition in a Small Lizard. J Exp Zool Part A Ecol Genet Physiol 2016;325(9):588–97.

20. Arcos-García JL, Ordaz JN, Grajales JG, et al. Body condition index in breeding black iguana females (Ctenosaura pectinata) in captivity. Rev la Fac Ciencias Agrar 2020;52(2):349–59.

21. Prebble JL, Shaw DJ, Meredith AL. Bodyweight and body condition score in rabbits on four different feeding regimes. J Small Anim Pract 2015;56(3):207–12.

22. Burton EJ, Newnham R, Bailey SJ, et al. Evaluation of a fast, objective tool for assessing body condition of budgerigars (Melopsittacus undulatus). J Anim Physiol Anim Nutr 2014;98(2):223–7.

23. Gimmel A, Öfner S, Liesegang A. Body condition scoring (BCS) in corn snakes (Pantherophis guttatus) and comparison to pre-existing body condition index (BCI) for snakes. J Anim Physiol Anim Nutr 2021;105(S2):24–8.

24. Nyeland J, Fox AD, Kahlert J, et al. Field methods to assess pectoral muscle mass in moulting geese. Wildlife Biol 2003;9(2):155–9.

25. Jayson S, Harding L, Michaels CJ, et al. Development of a body condition score for the mountain chicken frog (Leptodactylus fallax). Zoo Biol 2018;37(3): 196–205.

26. Rawski M, Józefiak D. Body condition scoring and obesity in captive African side-neck turtles (Pelomedusidae). Ann Anim Sci 2014;14(3):573–84.

27. Sweet H, Pearson AJ, Watson PJ, et al. A novel zoometric index for assessing body composition in adult rabbits. Vet Rec 2013;173(15):369.

28. Courcier EA, Mellor DJ, Pendlebury E, et al. Preliminary investigation to establish prevalence and risk factors for being overweight in pet rabbits in Great Britain. Vet Rec 2012;171(8):197.

29. Blem CR. Patterns of lipid storage and utilization in birds. Integr Comp Biol 1976;16(4):671–84.

30. Sion G, Watson MJ, Bouskila A. Measuring body condition of lizards: a comparison between non-invasive dual-energy X-ray absorptiometry, chemical fat extraction and calculated indices. Front Zool 2021;18(1):1–9.

31. Muscaritoli M, Anker SD, Argilés J, et al. Consensus definition of sarcopenia, cachexia and pre-cachexia: joint document elaborated by Special Interest Groups (SIG) " cachexia-anorexia in chronic wasting diseases" and " nutrition in geriatrics.". Clin Nutr 2010;29(2):154–9.

32. Fearon K, Strasser F, Anker SD, et al. Definition and classification of cancer cachexia: An international consensus. Lancet Oncol 2011;12(5):489–95.

33. Caporossi FS, Caporossi C, Borges Dock-Nascimento D, et al. Measurement of the thickness of the adductor pollicis muscle as a predictor of outcome in critically ill patients. Nutr Hosp 2012;27(2):490–5.

34. Freeman LM, Michel KE, Zanghi BM, et al. Evaluation of the use of muscle condition score and ultrasonographic measurements for assessment of muscle mass in dogs. Am J Vet Res 2019;80(6):595–600.

35. Michel KE, Anderson W, Cupp C, et al. Correlation of a feline muscle mass score with body composition determined by dual-energy X-ray absorptiometry. Br J Nutr 2011;106(S1):S57–9.

36. Humphreys J, De La Maza P, Hirsch S, et al. Muscle strength as a predictor of loss of functional status in hospitalized patients. Nutrition 2002;18(7–8):616–20.

37. Speakman JR, Van Acker A, Harper EJ. Age-related changes in the metabolism and body composition of three dog breeds and their relationship to life expectancy. Aging Cell 2003;2(5):265–75.

38. Susan EO. Critical care nutrition for exotic animals. J Exot Pet Med 2013;22(2): 163–77.

39. Beaufrère H. Nutrition and Fluid Therapy. In: Graham J, Doss G, Beaufrere H, editors. *Exotic animal Emergency and critical care medicine*. 5th edition. Hoboken, NJ: John Wiley & Sons, Inc; 2021. p. 503–17. https://doi.org/10.1002/9781119149262.ch46.

40. De Groof F, Joosten KFM, Janssen JAMJL, et al. Acute stress response in children with meningococcal sepsis: Important differences in the growth hormone/insulin-like growth factor I axis between nonsurvivors and survivors. J Clin Endocrinol Metab 2002;87(7):3118–24.

41. Mehta NM, Compher C. A.S.P.E.N. clinical guidelines: Nutrition support of the critically ill child. J Parenter Enter Nutr 2009;33(3):260–76.
42. McClave S a, Lowen CC, Kleber MJ, et al. Are patients fed appropriately according to their caloric requirements? J Parenter Enter Nutr 1998;22(6):375–81.
43. Elia M. Organ and tissue contribution to metabolic rate. In: Kinney J, Tucker H, editors. *Energy metabolism: tissue Determinants and cellular Corollaries*. New York: Raven Press; 1992. p. 61–80.
44. Müller MJ, Bosy-Westphal A, Kutzner D, et al. Metabolically active components of fat free mass (FFM) and resting energy expenditure (REE) in humans. Forum Nutr 2003;56(3):301–3.
45. Das SK, Saltzman E, McCrory MA, et al. Energy expenditure is very high in extremely obese women. J Nutr 2004;134(6):1412–6.
46. Bermingham EN, Thomas DG, Morris PJ, et al. Energy requirements of adult cats. Br J Nutr 2010;103(8):1083–93.
47. Ahmed J, Khan LUR, Khan S, et al. Refeeding syndrome: A literature review. Gastroenterol Res Pract 2011;2011.
48. Go HK, Lee SJ, Cho IG, et al. Changes of blood Mg2+ and K+ after starvation during molting in laying hens. J Vet Clin 2011;28(6):581–5.
49. Cook S, Whitby E, Elias N, et al. Retrospective evaluation of refeeding syndrome in cats: 11 cases (2013–2019). J Feline Med Surg 2021;23(10):883–91.
50. De Voe RS. Nutritional support of reptile patients. Vet Clin North Am - Exot Anim Pract. 2014;17(2):249–61.
51. Bookbinder L, Schott HC. Refeeding syndrome in a miniature donkey. J Vet Emerg Crit Care 2021;31(5):668–73.
52. Lakshmanan R, Senthilkumar K, Balagangatharathilagar M, et al. Emergency and critical care in green iguana (Iguana iguana): a case report. Int J Sci Environ Technol 2020;9(3):447–50. Available at: www.ijset.net.
53. Mehanna HM, Moledina J, Travis J. Refeeding syndrome: What it is, and how to prevent and treat it. BMJ 2008;336(7659):1495–8.
54. Puchalska P, Crawford PA. Multi-dimensional roles of ketone bodies in fuel metabolism, signaling, and therapeutics. Cell Metab 2017;25(2):262–84.
55. McGarry JD, Foster DW. Ketogenesis and cholesterol synthesis in normal and neoplastic tissues of the rat. J Biol Chem 1969;244(15):4251–6.
56. Cohen P, Stark E. Hepatic ketogenesis and ketolysis in different species. J Biol Chem 1938;126(1):97–107.
57. Sampson J. Ketosis in Domestic animals: clinical and Experimental Observations. Urbana, IL: University of Illinois Agricultural Experiment Station; 1947. https://doi.org/10.5962/bhl.title.16684.
58. Lindholm C, Altimiras J, Lees J. Measuring ketones in the field: rapid and reliable measures of β-hydroxybutyrate in birds. Ibis 2019;161(1):205–10.
59. Price ER. The physiology of lipid storage and use in reptiles. Biol Rev 2017; 92(3):1406–26.
60. Hildebrandt MA, Hoffmann C, Sherrill-Mix SA, et al. High-Fat Diet Determines the Composition of the Murine Gut Microbiome Independently of Obesity. Gastroenterology 2009;137(5):1716–24.e2.
61. Duan Y, Zeng L, Zheng C, et al. Inflammatory links between high fat diets and diseases. Front Immunol 2018;9(NOV):1–10.
62. National Research Council. Nutrient requirements of laboratory animals. 4th edition. Washington, DC: The National Academies Press; 1995. https://doi.org/10.17226/4758.

63. National Research Council. Nutrient requirements of poultry. 9th edition. Washington, DC: The National Academies Press; 1994. https://doi.org/10.17226/2114.

64. National Research Council (NRC). Nutrient requirements of dogs and cats. Washington, DC: National Academies Press; 2006. https://doi.org/10.17226/10668.

65. Watkins BA. Importance of essential fatty acids and their derivatives in poultry. J Nutr 1991;121(9):1475–85.

66. Lauritzen L, Brambilla P, Mazzocchi A, et al. DHA effects in brain development and function. Nutrients 2016;8(1):1–17.

67. Pawlosky R, Barnes a, Salem N Jr. Essential fatty acid metabolism in the feline: relationship between liver and brain production of long-chain polyunsaturated fatty acids. J Lipid Res 1994;35(11):2032–40. Available at: http://www.ncbi.nlm.nih.gov/entrez/query.fcgi?cmd=Retrieve&db=PubMed&dopt=Citation&list_uids=7868981.

68. Morris JG, Rogers QR. Arginine: An essential amino acid for the cat. J Nutr 1978;108(12):1944–53.

69. Deshmukh DR, Shope TC. Arginine requirement and ammonia toxicity in ferrets. J Nutr 1983;113(8):1664–7.

70. Ziegler F, Ollivier JM, Cynober L, et al. Efficiency of enteral nitrogen support in surgical patients: Small peptides v non-degraded proteins. Gut 1990;31(11):1277–83.

71. Rooze S, Namane SA, Beretta X, et al. Is a semi-elemental diet better than a polymeric diet after congenital heart surgery? Eur J Pediatr 2020;179(3):423–30.

72. Finco DR, Brown SA, Crowell WA, et al. Effects of dietary phosphorus and protein in dogs with chronic renal failure. Am J Vet Res 1992;53(12):2264–71.

73. Finco DR, Brown Sa, Brown Ca, et al. Protein and calorie effects on progression of induced chronic renal failure in cats. Am J Vet Res 1998;59(5):575–82.

74. Burkholder WJ, Lees GE, LeBlanc AK, et al. Diet modulates proteinuria in heterozygous female dogs with X-linked hereditary nephropathy. J Vet Intern Med 2009;18(2):165–75.

75. Watford M. Glutamine and glutamate: Nonessential or essential amino acids? Anim Nutr 2015;1(3):119–22.

76. Fürst P, Albers S, Stehle P. Evidence for a nutritional need for glutamine in catabolic patients. Kidney Int Suppl 1989;27:S287–92. Available at: http://www.ncbi.nlm.nih.gov/pubmed/2517677.

77. Singer P, Blaser AR, Berger MM, et al. ESPEN guideline on clinical nutrition in the intensive care unit. Clin Nutr 2019;38(1):48–79.

78. Winternitz WW, Lattanzi WE. Liver glycogen reserves in experimental diabetic ketosis. Endocrinology 1956;58(2):232–42.

79. Warriss PD, Kestin SC, Brown SN, et al. Depletion of glycogen reserves in fasting broiler chickens. Br Poult Sci 1988;29(1):149–54.

80. Morris JG, Trudell J, Pencovic T. Carbohydrate digestion by the domestic cat (Felis catus). Br J Nutr 1977;37(3):365–73.

81. Meyer H, Kienzle E. Dietary protein and carbohydrates: relationship to clinical disease. Purina International Symposium 1991;15:13–26.

82. Faustino EV, Apkon M. Persistent hyperglycemia in critically ill children. J Pediatr 2005;146(1):30–4.

83. Zelihic E, Poneleit B, Siegmund T, et al. Hyperglycemia in emergency patients – prevalence and consequences. Eur J Emerg Med 2015;22(3):181–7.

84. Gore DC, Chinkes D, Heggers J, et al. Association of hyperglycemia with increased mortality after severe burn injury. J Trauma Acute Care Surg 2001; 51(3):540–4.
85. Queau Y, Larsen JA, Kass PH, et al. Factors associated with adverse outcomes during parenteral nutrition administration in dogs and cats. J Vet Intern Med 2011;25(3):446–52.
86. Chan DL, Freeman LM, Labato MA, et al. Retrospective evaluation of partial parenteral nutrition in dogs and cats. J Vet Intern Med 2002;16(4):440–5.
87. Heilig CW, Concepcion LA, Riser BL, et al. Overexpression of glucose transporters in rat mesangial cells cultured in a normal glucose milieu mimics the diabetic phenotype. J Clin Invest 1995;96(4):1802–14.
88. Kaiser N, Sasson S, Feener EP, et al. Differential regulation of glucose transport and transporters by glucose in vascular endothelial and smooth muscle cells. Diabetes 1993;42(1):80–9.
89. Dimitrakoudis D, Vranic M, Klip A. Effects of hyperglycemia on glucose transporters of the muscle: Use of the renal glucose reabsorption inhibitor phlorizin to control glycemia. J Am Soc Nephrol 1992;3(5):1078–91.
90. Van den Berghe G, Wouters P, Weekers F, et al. Intensive insulin therapy in critically ill patients. N Engl J Med 2001;345(19):1359–67.
91. Krinsley JS. Effect of an intensive glucose management protocol on the mortality of critically ill adult patients. Mayo Clin Proc 2004;79(8):992–1000.
92. Torre DM, DeLaforcade AM, Chan DL. Incidence and clinical relevance of hyperglycemia in critically ill dogs. J Vet Intern Med 2007;21(5):971–5.
93. Ray CC, Callahan-Clark J, Beckel NF, et al. The prevalence and significance of hyperglycemia in hospitalized cats. J Vet Emerg Crit Care 2009;19(4):347–51.
94. Grant K. Rodent nutrition: Digestive comparisons of 4 common rodent species. Vet Clin North Am - Exot Anim Pract 2014;17(3):471–83.
95. National Research Council. Nutrient requirements of rabbits. Washington, DC: The National Academies Press; 1977. https://doi.org/10.17226/35.
96. Singh AK, Kim WK. Effects of dietary fiber on nutrients utilization and gut health of poultry: A review of challenges and opportunities. Animals 2021;11(1):1–18.
97. Wehrle BA, German DP. Reptilian digestive efficiency: Past, present, and future. Comp Biochem Physiol -Part A Mol Integr Physiol. 2023;277:111369.
98. Gow AG, Else R, Evans H, et al. Hypovitaminosis D in dogs with inflammatory bowel disease and hypoalbuminaemia. J Small Anim Pract 2011;52(8):411–8.
99. Jaffey JA, Backus RC, McDaniel KM, et al. Serum Vitamin D concentrations in hospitalized critically ill dogs. PLoS One 2018;13(3):1–15.
100. Sato PH, Grahn IV. Administration of isolated chicken l-gulonolactone oxidase to guinea pigs evokes ascorbic acid synthetic capacity. Arch Biochem Biophys 1981;210(2):609–16.
101. Palmieri B, Vadalà M, Laurino C. Nutrition in wound healing: investigation of the molecular mechanisms, a narrative review. J Wound Care 2019;28(10):683–93.
102. Guo S, DiPietro LA. Critical review in oral biology & medicine: Factors affecting wound healing. J Dent Res 2010;89(3):219–29.
103. Carr AC, Rosengrave PC, Bayer S, et al. Hypovitaminosis C and vitamin C deficiency in critically ill patients despite recommended enteral and parenteral intakes. Crit Care 2017;21(1):1–10.
104. Long CL, Maull KI, Krishnan RS, et al. Ascorbic acid dynamics in the seriously ill and injured. J Surg Res 2003;109(2):144–8.
105. Nandi BK, Majumder AK, Subramanian N, et al. Effects of Large Doses of Vitamin C in Guinea Pigs and Rats. J Nutr 1973;103(12):1688–95.

106. Kraus VB, Huebner JL, Stabler T, et al. Ascorbic acid increases the severity of spontaneous knee osteoarthritis in a guinea pig model. Arthritis Rheum 2004; 50(6):1822–31.

107. Kim MH, Choi MK. Seven Dietary Minerals (Ca, P, Mg, Fe, Zn, Cu, and Mn) and Their Relationship with Blood Pressure and Blood Lipids in Healthy Adults with Self-Selected Diet. Biol Trace Elem Res 2013;153(1–3):69–75.

108. Cray C. Reference Intervals in Avian and Exotic Hematology. Vet Clin North Am - Exot Anim Pract. 2015;18(1):105–16.

109. Harr KE. Diagnostic value of biochemistry. In: *Clinical avian medicine*2. Palm Beach, FL: Spix Publishing, Inc; 2011. p. 611–29.

110. Ozawa S, Thomson A, Petritz O. Safety and efficacy of oral mirtazapine in New Zealand White rabbits (Oryctolagus cuniculus). J Exot Pet Med 2022;40:16–20.

111. Scagnelli A, Titel C, Doss G, et al. Effects of midazolam and lorazepam on food intake in budgerigars (Melopsittacus undulatus). J Exot Pet Med 2022;41:42–5.

112. Martel A, Berg C, Doss G, et al. Effects of Midazolam on Food Intake in Budgerigars (Melopsittacus undulatus). J Avian Med Surg 2022;36(1). https://doi.org/10.1647/20-00096.

113. Whittington JK. Esophagostomy feeding tube use and placement in exotic pets. J Exot Pet Med 2013;22(2):178–91.

114. Bernstein IL. Development of food aversions during illness. Proc Nutr Soc 1994; 53(1):131–7.

115. Forman MA, Steiner JM, Armstrong PJ, et al. ACVIM consensus statement on pancreatitis in cats. J Vet Intern Med 2021;35(2):703–23.

116. Dogterom GJ, van Hof MW. Attenuation of neophobia and conditioned taste aversion in the rabbit. Behav Brain Res 1988;28(3):253–7.

117. Rabin BM, Hunt WA. Relationship between vomiting and taste aversion learning in the ferret: studies with ionizing radiation, lithium chloride, and amphetamine. Behav Neural Biol 1992;58(2):83–93.

118. Mason JR, Reidinger RF. Observational learning of food aversions in Red-winged Blackbirds (Agelaius phoeniceus). Auk 1982;99(3):548–54.

119. Ward-Fear G, Thomas J, Webb JK, et al. Eliciting conditioned taste aversion in lizards: Live toxic prey are more effective than scent and taste cues alone. Integr Zool 2017;12(2):112–20.

120. Paradis S, Cabanac M. Flavor aversion learning induced by lithium chloride in reptiles but not in amphibians. Behav Processes 2004;67(1):11–8.

121. Garcia J, Hankins WG, Rusiniak KW. Behavioral Regulation of the Milieu Interne in Man and Rat. Science 1974;185(4154):824–31.

122. Powers LV. Common Procedures in Psittacines. Vet Clin North Am Exot Anim Pract 2006;9(2):287–302.

123. Briscoe JA, Latney L, Heinze CR. Nutritional support in exotic pet species. In: Chan D, editor. *Nutritional Management of hospitalized small animals*. West Sussex, UK: John Wiley & Sons, Ltd; 2015. p. 234–46. https://doi.org/10.1002/9781119052951.ch25.

124. Papavramidis T, Kaidoglou K, Grosomanidis V, et al. Ann 2009;22(4):268–74. Available at: http://www.annalsgastro.gr/index.php/annalsgastro/article/view/770.

125. Hernandez G, Velasco N, Wainstein C, et al. Gut mucosal atrophy after a short enteral fasting period in critically ill patients. J Crit Care 1999;14(2):73–7.

126. Kozeniecki M, Fritzshall R. Enteral Nutrition for Adults in the Hospital Setting. Nutr Clin Pract 2015;30(5):634–51.

127. Mihai R, Florescu IP, Coroiu V, et al. In vitro biocompatibility testing of some synthetic polymers used for the achievement of nervous conduits. J Med Life 2011; 4(3):250–5.

128. Wallace T, Steward D. Gastric Tube Use and Care in the NICU. Newborn Infant Nurs Rev 2014;14(3):103–8.

129. Peter CS, Wiechers C, Bohnhorst B, et al. Influence of nasogastric tubes on gastroesophageal reflux in preterm infants: A multiple intraluminal impedance study. J Pediatr 2002;141(2):277–9.

130. Chen CN, Wu MS, Lien GS, et al. Influence of replacing percutaneous endoscopic gastrostomy for nasogastric tube feeding on gastroesophageal reflux disease with erosive esophagitis. Adv Dig Med 2016;3(2):49–55.

131. Yu MK, Freeman LM, Heinze CR, et al. Comparison of complication rates in dogs with nasoesophageal versus nasogastric feeding tubes. J Vet Emerg Crit Care 2013;23(3):300–4.

132. Ross S. Utilization of Feeding Tubes in the Management of Feline Chronic Kidney Disease. Vet Clin North Am - Small Anim Pract. 2016;46(6):1099–114.

133. Cavanaugh RP, Kovak JR, Fischetti AJ, et al. Evaluation of surgically placed gastrojejunostomy feeding tubes in critically ill dogs. J Am Vet Med Assoc 2008;232(3):380–8.

134. Furthner E, Kowalewski MP, Torgerson P, et al. Verifying the placement and length of feeding tubes in canine and feline neonates. BMC Vet Res 2021; 17(1):1–12.

135. Johnson PA, Mann FA, Dodam J, et al. Capnographic documentation of nasoesophageal and nasogastric feeding tube placement in dogs. J Vet Emerg Crit Care 2002;12(4):227–33.

136. Kindopp AS, Drover JW, Heyland DK. Capnography confirms correct feeding tube placement in intensive care unit patients. Can J Anesth 2001;48(7):705–10.

137. Bullen LE. Nutrition for Pocket Pets (Ferrets, Rabbits, and Rodents). Vet Clin North Am - Small Anim Pract. 2021;51(3):583–604.

138. Johnson-Delaney CA. Ferret nutrition. Vet Clin North Am - Exot Anim Pract. 2014; 17(3):449–70.

139. Donoghue S, McKeown S. Nutrition of captive reptiles. Vet Clin North Am Exot Anim Pract 1999;2(1):69–91.

Interpretation of Serum Analytes for Nutritional Evaluation

Kathleen E. Sullivan, MS, PhD*, Alyxandra Swanhall, BS,
Shannon Livingston, MSc

KEYWORDS

- Micronutrient • Vitamin • Mineral • Normality • Imbalance • Blood

KEY POINTS

- Diagnostic connections between serum micronutrients and dietary status should be made with caution, rather than an assumption of direct cause/effect. There are many serum changes that do not warrant diet alteration.
- Most of the micronutrients interact with each other, both in the diet and in the body, which will influence their activity.
- Normality, as equated to health, in serum nutrients across exotic species is not a uniform range. Serum reference ranges for exotic species do not necessarily convey normality.

INTRODUCTION

Nutrition is a fundamental pillar of animal welfare and challenging in its impact on maintaining optimal health. A correct balance of macro and micronutrients in the diet as well as considerations of physical form and feeding will sustain optimal physiologic processes throughout life. This leads to three fundamentally difficult questions that often cannot be directly known—What is the correct nutrient balance for your animal? How do you evaluate optimal health in terms of nutrition? How can blood testing aid in this evaluation?

The place to begin looking at nutrient balance will be ensuring energy requirements are met by the diet macronutrients: protein, carbohydrate, and fat. Evaluating energy requirements can be estimated using published energy equations, but an animal's actual energy status must be refined by assessing the diet's impact on body weight and body condition over time. Once energetic needs are met, further evaluation of the diet consists of calculating whether nutrient composition of the diet as consumed (rather than as offered) is meeting the estimated requirements of the animal.

Disney's Animals, Science and Environment, 1180 North Savannah Circle, Lake Buena Vista, FL 32830, USA
* Corresponding author:
E-mail address: Kathleen.E.Sullivan@disney.com

Vet Clin Exot Anim 27 (2024) 135–154
https://doi.org/10.1016/j.cvex.2023.08.004
1094-9194/24/© 2023 Elsevier Inc. All rights reserved.
vetexotic.theclinics.com

Unfortunately, published nutrient targets can be lacking for many exotic species. Domestic model requirements may not be ideal for all exotics due to domestic breeding for production and species' physiologic differences. However, domestic model requirements give starting context for nutrient evaluation. Investigating diet digestibility in the species can also improve the accuracy of the overall assessment. Are they able to digest and use the nutrients in the diet offered? And how can blood testing, a commonly used diagnostic tool, also be used to delve deeper?

There are many guides on interpretation of blood chemistry in relation to nutritional issues in cats and dogs as well as domestic livestock. Excellent discussions of trace mineral serum interpretation in these domestic species also exist in the literature.[1–4] This article, however, focuses on the challenges of serum mineral and vitamin interpretations across exotic species and identifies caveats involving knowledge gaps. Analyte concentrations will commonly be compared with reported reference ranges, but it is important to recognize that these can vary by species, and in some cases, may not be supported by strong data from healthy animals. No matter the serum analyte measured, all diagnostic connections between "low" or "high" serum concentrations and clinical signs should be made with caution. The aim of this article, therefore, is not to provide an exhaustive list of all potential reference values for serum/plasma micronutrient biochemistry across exotic species, but rather to highlight considerations in interpretation and further nutritional understanding.

Commonly, initial diagnostic blood testing focuses on a CBC (complete blood count/hematology) and blood chemistry profile. However, further serum vitamin and mineral analysis may be warranted in particular cases. Whether to pursue these additional serum nutrient analyses depends on the clinical question at hand and whether nutrition may play a role: in prevention, as an associated causative agent and/or in management strategy. It is important to remember, however, that although diet certainly impacts circulating nutrient concentrations, the relationship between serum analyte concentrations and clinical presentation may not be direct, as "cause and effect," due to various metabolic factors affecting digestion and absorption.

Choosing a Laboratory

Although CBC and blood chemistry panels are fairly ubiquitous across laboratories, with well-calibrated machines and trained personnel, the accuracy and reliability of serum mineral and vitamin analysis can vary between laboratories. Analysis for specific amino acids, fatty acids, or micronutrients in blood should be performed at a reliable commercial laboratory that regularly works with animal samples and ideally has experience with samples from exotic species. There are several excellently regarded laboratories in the United States, many associated with a veterinary college but also some commercial. Once a laboratory is selected, it is worthwhile to reach out and ask a few questions, to plan in advance for taking, handling, and shipping samples and interpreting results.

- What sample type, whole blood versus plasma versus serum, would be best for the type of analysis desired? What blood tube should be used for evaluating the micronutrient in question, as different tube coatings/additives may interfere with analysis?
- Does the sample require special handling and/or shipping procedures, such as protection from light or ship overnight on dry ice to the laboratory?
- What is the analytical method being used, for example, high permonce liquid chromatography (HPLC) or liquid chromatography with tandem mass spectrometry (LC-MS-MS) or enzyme-linked immunosorbent assay (ELISA) kit? Does the

laboratory have a quality assurance program and expertise in this particular area?

- For mineral analysis, was the sample analyzed via atomic absorption or inductively coupled plasma mass spectrometry (ICP-MS)? In this case, both options may get reliable results but could have unit differences to consider.
- What units will the results be reported in and are those comparable to reported reference ranges? Molar values are not equivalent to standard units for most nutrients, so if help is needed with unit conversion, reach out to the laboratory for assistance.

The more you know about your sample and the analysis, the more confidence you will have interpreting your results. Inevitably, however, there will be a time when variable or questionable results arise. This is when developing a relationship with a laboratory that you trust, one that is transparent, open to communication, and committed to troubleshooting, will help tremendously. Questionable results can be a consequence of your own sample handling and processing, the laboratory technique used, and/or the laboratory staff's level of experience processing exotic samples. For example, not every laboratory that measures serum vitamin D performs the analysis with the same technical caliber or is able to measure vitamin E when circulating concentrations are low. Likewise, not all laboratories perform mineral analysis with the same analytical method, impacting results reporting. Therefore, if your serum result varies markedly from either what you expect, a reported reference range, or a previous measurement taken, first verify the units are comparable and then reach out to the laboratory to troubleshoot.

Understanding the Impact of Serum Analytes on Nutrition

The connection between serum analytes and nutrients entering the body is not always straightforward, as metabolism regulates the movement of these chemicals as they incorporate and react, changing as they travel. The interplay of nutrients because they are absorbed across membranes, stored in organs, and exist in circulation, and their impact on health is complicated. Our focus here is on the lesser understood micronutrients; however, entire texts have been written on interpretation of hematology and basic blood chemistry panels, including liver and kidney function indicators as well as macronutrient references (ie, glucose, cholesterol, triglycerides, total protein).

Blood chemistry panels cover a range of nutrient-related parameters, including electrolytes, total protein, glucose, cholesterol, triglycerides, calcium (Ca), magnesium (Mg), and phosphorus (P). You can also gain insight on excess fat in circulation from a lipemia index. Electrolytes, including sodium (Na), potassium, and chloride, are snapshots of current electrolyte status so should be considered in light of the animal's current health and fed status. Creatinine is an indicator of hydration status and linked to glomerular filtration rate and protein intake.[5] There are excellent reviews on these analytes in several places, including Cornell's veterinary reference Web site (https://eclinpath.com/chemistry/).

Changes in hematology are strongly connected to iron (Fe) status; zinc (Zn), copper (Cu), cobalt (Co), and other micronutrients may also play into red blood cell formation and proliferation as well as cell-mediated immune system function. Anemia specifically has many underlying causes, including Fe deficiency, B-12 deficiency potentially relating to Co, Cu deficiency, folate deficiency, and the anemia of chronic disease, among others.[6] However, again, you cannot assume causation based on serum results alone, as animal age, health and reproductive status, the diet, medication, and supplementation regimen, and so forth may influence these micronutrient parameters and the disease state itself.

Considering Reference Ranges and Normality

When interpreting serum analytes for exotic species, acknowledging the animals' natural history, including diet, and using normal reference ranges for domestic species are great first steps for consideration. Some published reference ranges for exotic species are available, but most lack a proven and established understanding of normality. Commonly, misinterpretations can stem from reference ranges reported by commercial laboratories for exotic species. Laboratory-reported reference ranges often are based on a compilation of samples they have analyzed, with inadequate distinction between sample results from healthy or sick animals; no consideration of variable diet histories; and no qualification as to whether animals were wild, rehabilitating, or under human care. In some cases, this reference summary is helpful as a guide; however, if there is a large standard error, creating a wide range of "normality"; more closely investigate what "healthy" means within that parameter. For example, if a whole population of chameleons has low vitamin A compared with mammalian references, does it mean that a low vitamin A is also normal for chameleons? One could argue that yes, low serum vitamin A could also be normal for chameleons, but is a low serum vitamin A necessary for the species to function optimally. One could then argue that no, low serum vitamin A should not be expected because chameleons have a carnivorous diet.

Knowing Your Diet History

In clinical veterinary practice of any kind, understanding what food is consumed by an animal is critical to assessment of welfare and can potentially alter a diagnosis and/or treatment regimen. An accurate diet history can be challenging to obtain, as it is generally based on caretaker records or in some cases, memories. However, once you have this information, even an estimate of intake can give insights to help make connections with blood testing results. Although commercial complete feeds are designed to be balanced and meet minimal requirements for domestic species, many additional food items from produce to supplements can be offered and can unbalance an animals' diet. Similarly, the true diet consumed by the animal, rather than the one offered or prescribed, dictates nutritional balance. Micronutrients are not always impacted by the diet to a point of clear imbalance, but without knowledge of diet provided, analyzed serum micronutrient concentrations cannot be fully understood.

When assessing the diet, use publicly available resources on food nutritional content from trusted sources, including the United States Department of Agriculture (USDA's) helpful resource (https://fdc.nal.usda.gov/) and feed composition databases such as Dairy One Forage Laboratory's (https://apps.dairyone.com/feedcomposition/). Nutrient profiles for many exotic commercial complete diets are unavailable, however, on these platforms. Manufacturers will supply the average nutritional content of their pelleted feeds, some including more information than others. If limited information is provided, it may be worthwhile to analyze the feed further to understand starch, sugar, mineral, and vitamin contents; often these components are not reported by the manufacturer and have the potential to impact serum analytes. However, unless an issue with the feed is suspected, it is likely unnecessary to invest in diet laboratory analysis; instead, communicate with feed companies to learn more about the nutritional composition of their products, especially if labeling is unclear and/or if knowledge of a particular nutrient concentration may help diagnosis. It is important to remember that formulations are often proprietary, and there is no legal obligation for feed companies to share that information.

DISCUSSION

Although serum or plasma levels of minerals and vitamins may give insight into feeding, this assumption is not uniform. Detecting biochemical changes in fluids and tissues of animals that correspond with clinical and pathologic consequences are often dependent on the nutrient in question. For the purposes of this article, the minerals and vitamins discussed in detail are the most commonly analyzed.

The early detection of mineral imbalances is tied to whether the mineral has a large storage pool within the body.[4] Classification of minerals as Type 1 (Ca, Co, Cu, Fe, and I), where bodies can store a larger pool when the diet provides more than animals require, or Type 2 (K, Mg, Mn, Na, P, S, and Se) which have minimal storage, can help delineate expectations on how deficiency or toxicity occur.[7] However, skepticism is encouraged when analytes seem higher or lower than a reference range for the species in question. There are many exceptions to a clear diagnosis of nutrient—dependent deficiency. For example, a low serum Zn value in a sick rabbit is more likely a product of stress than dietary deficiency.

Vitamins function in metabolism in five general ways: as coenzymes, in redox reduction/oxidation chemistry as donors and acceptors of electrons, antioxidants, hormones, and effectors of gene transcription.[3] Serum assessment of vitamins is generally a direct assessment of nutritional status and is impacted by the nutrient's form and bioavailability in diet. Only vitamins D_3, niacin, and vitamin C can be made by the body, though there are exceptions to all three across species—for example, niacin provided only by tryptophan conversion does not meet biological needs in many cat species.[3,8] Changes in vitamin status can be impacted not only by diet availability but by effective supply of the vitamin in the body or increased needs and use. Fat soluble vitamins have more capacity for storage than water soluble vitamins.[2] Storage of food items can impact vitamin stability, such as the destruction of thiamin and vitamin E across time in frozen fish.[9]

Although understanding total vitamin and mineral balance within the body can be daunting, knowing when to connect serum analytes to an animals' diet or not has more guideposts.

CALCIUM AND PHOSPHORUS

Calcium (Ca) and phosphorus (P) are considered macro-minerals as they are present in larger quantities in the body. Ca serves multiple functions as the major component of bone, nerve conduction, muscle contraction, and a variety of cell signaling.[4] Serum levels of Ca and P are tightly regulated to maintain relatively consistent concentrations via several metabolic pathways involving parathyroid hormone (PTH), sex hormones, and renal health.[10–13] To some extent, dietary intake of Ca, P, Na, and vitamin D also can impact circulating Ca and P.

In mammals, dietary Ca intake may result in a transient elevation of serum Ca if the sample was obtained closely after the animal has eaten.[14,15] In both birds and reptiles, however, dietary intake directly influences serum Ca.[10,16] Understanding when the animal last ate, therefore, aids in interpretation of serum results. Further, the amount of Ca absorbed from the diet and relative serum Ca concentrations can be influenced by total body stores, growth, reproduction, and renal health.[17,18] For example, when circulating Ca is low, dietary absorption is upregulated to maintain serum concentrations.[4] As another example, serum Ca levels can be significantly elevated in both birds and reptiles during egg laying/ovulation.[10,12,16] Differences in species physiology may also play a role; rabbits have both active transport and passive diffusion of dietary Ca that directly impacts serum Ca and results in concentrations 30% to 50% greater than those reported for other mammals.[18,19]

For most species, the dietary ratio of Ca to P (or Ca:P) should be minimally 1:1 to 2:1, to maintain a similar desired ratio in the serum.[10,20] At certain times in an animal's life or for species where the dietary need for Ca is greater, a higher dietary Ca:P may be necessary. Differences in physiology may also come into play; for example, research in elasmobranchs indicates that these cartilaginous fish may regularly have serum Ca:P closer to 3:1.[13] In addition, the dietary contribution of P, Na, and vitamin D can impact circulating Ca. Diets rich in P, such as those often fed to insectivorous reptiles, result in lower intestinal absorption of Ca, reducing circulating Ca concentrations. This will then stimulate PTH secretion, resulting in bone resorption to support circulating Ca levels.[21] Diets providing high Na concentrations result in greater renal excretion of Ca, which may reduce circulating Ca concentrations. Diets both rich and poor in vitamin D can impact circulating Ca and P.[4] High dietary vitamin D can result in both hypercalcemia and hyperphosphatemia in several species,[10,16,18,22] whereas low dietary vitamin D is associated with reduced serum P in tenrecs.[23]

It is also important to consider how serum Ca is being evaluated. Total serum Ca can fluctuate widely due to the aforementioned mechanisms (eg, egg laying), so instead, using ionized Ca provides a better measure of true Ca status.[10–12,24–26] Unreliable serum Ca results may be encountered if the wrong blood collection tube was used, the sample was hemolyzed, contaminated with bacteria, or inadvertently diluted, or if the animal is alkalotic, causing increased Ca-protein binding and reduced free Ca.[10,14]

Dietary P and its relative intestinal absorption may influence serum P, but various species-dependent factors influencing serum P, such as circadian rhythm, recycling from salivary secretions, bone dynamics, and milk and egg production, complicate interpretation.[4] Absorption of dietary P increases, often with corresponding serum elevation, when serum vitamin D is elevated, body P is low, or the demand for P is high, such as in growth. Younger animals may have normal elevations in serum P during periods of bone growth.[12,18]

The majority of P in foods such as nuts, seeds, beans, legumes, and grains, can be found as phytic acid or phytate, a complex of six P molecules. Dietary phytate binds minerals such as Ca, Zn, and Fe, rendering all (P included) unavailable for absorption without microbial influence. Microbes produce the non-mammalian enzyme phytase, allowing species ranging from ruminants to hind-gut fermenters such as horses, to use phytate P.[27,28] It is important, therefore, to consider the potential phytate content of a diet if clinical symptoms of deficiency seem in minerals commonly bound to phytate.

MAGNESIUM

Magnesium (Mg) functions in stabilizing a wide array of enzymatic reactions with the majority of body Mg held in bone and soft tissue. Only about 0.3% of total body Mg is found in serum, making it a poor indicator of body status, except in deficiency.[29] Mg levels in circulation are generally kept to a tight range (most mammalian reference ranges are close to 2 mg/dL). The kidneys regulate Mg excretion in direct correlation to intake avoiding toxicity concerns.[30]

Low serum Mg will lead to low serum Ca; as Mg is needed for PTH secretion, which regulates Ca metabolism in both the bones and kidney. Treating the Mg deficiency with supplementation or rebalancing the diet will be needed to reverse the low

Ca.[31] Serum Mg can be influenced by dietary antagonists including high potassium, phytate, and fibers. Although supplementation for low Mg can be considered, make sure a total diet assessment is performed, as balanced herbivorous diets should have multiple sources of Mg. The best sources of Mg are vegetables, leafy greens, grains, and legumes. Hypomagnesaemia as tetany (neuromuscular disorder with muscle rigidity) has been shown to occur across species. In grazing herbivores, pastures fertilized with high-potassium chemicals can lead to tetany.[32]

IRON

Iron (Fe) is necessary in the body for oxygen transport, DNA synthesis, and as a cofactor in many biological reactions, using stored Fe to address both acute and chronic Fe needs. This creates a need for well-balanced Fe metabolism, to absorb enough to not deplete stores, whereas not creating an excess of potentially dangerous Fe within the body. Interpreting serum Fe is complicated by species differences in Fe homeostasis. Serum Fe can reflect dietary influences, but a wide range of circulating Fe may be acceptable for function within the body. Serum Fe ranges in reptiles are generally lower than mammals. Fe is regulated via absorption, with the majority in the body pool residing as part of the reticuloendothelial cycle, or the creation and breakdown of red blood cells. Assuming no genetic abnormalities, most animals should be able to absorb the 1% to 2% of dietary Fe they need to replenish the minor endogenous losses.[33] Hence, most Fe fed to healthy animals is not absorbed. Fe does not have a documented route of internal excretion across species. Fe content is highest in animal products but also present in legumes and leafy vegetables.

High serum Fe is dangerous due to cytotoxic reactions of free Fe creating free oxygen radicals. The majority of Fe is bound or carried within proteins to avoid this hazard. Fe intoxication from diet is possible, with or without the genetic forms of hemochromatosis, with more than 30 species including toucans, starlings, lemurs, red deer, uakari, and fruit bats demonstrating Fe overloading under human care.[34] When there are concerns of high bioavailable Fe intake, especially in an Fe-sensitive species, it is recommended to assess transferrin saturation, or how saturated Fe transporters are in the blood, as serum Fe does not always elevate immediately with Fe loading.[4,35] More than 60% transferrin saturation, for all species, indicates that there are risks for oxidative damage and negative repercussions in the body.[36] Ferritin, an Fe storage protein, is a better measure of body stores across time than serum Fe, which provides more of a snapshot.[34,35,37] Ferritin is a species-specific acute-phase protein, though it has a strongly conserved structure across species allowing assay crossover.[37,38] Kansas State Veterinary Diagnostic Laboratory provides commercial assays validated for ferritin for diverse species including canines, rhinos, dolphins, felines, and equids.

Fe deficiency is often reflected hematologically as forms of anemia. However, anemias from a lack of dietary Fe differ from those associated with chronic disease, infection, or general malnutrition.[4] Fe absorption may be antagonized by other minerals, inflammation, lack of stomach acid, or the presence of phytate, oxalates, or polyphenols. Although increasing dietary Fe may help, adequate vitamin B12, Cu, and vitamin C in the diet are also needed to ensure utilization and uptake of Fe in the body. For example, vitamin C fed in conjunction with Fe increases Fe absorption by reducing its absorbable state to cross the gut wall.[39] Heme Fe from meat sources avoids gut transporter regulation, allowing easier absorption; therefore, carnivores with anemias are less likely to stem from dietary deficiencies. Plant sources of Fe are often poorly bioavailable due to phytate binding. Legumes, such as clover, alfalfa, and soy, tend to have high levels of Fe stored in plant ferritin that also avoid gut transporter regulation, serving to help combat deficiencies or contribute to Fe loading in excess.[40,41]

ZINC

Zinc (Zn) is one of the most abundant microminerals in the body critical to cellular function and comprises numerous enzymes, including superoxide dismutase.[1] Zn regulates growth, appetite, and immune health.[4] Natural dietary sources of Zn include meat, fish, crustaceans, beans, nuts, whole grains, and some legumes.[42,43] Dietary Zn absorption and excretion are closely linked with total body status; for example, an increase in dietary Zn, when deficiency is not present, will lead to a decrease in intestinal Zn absorption and an increase in fecal excretion.[44]

Most animals have a high Zn tolerance, so toxicity is rare except in cases of excessive intake. Zn deficiency is more common and occurs often in relation to high levels of phytate and Ca in the diet. In nonruminant species, dietary Zn bound to phytates is unavailable because there is no mechanism for releasing the Zn to be available for absorption, ultimately leading to Zn deficiency. Zn supplementation, or providing supplemental dietary phytase, can reverse the mineral deficiency.[45]

Serum Zn is influenced by inflammation, hypoalbuminemia (two-thirds of serum Zn is bound to albumin), and improper handling.[1] Serum and plasma samples can be used for evaluating biochemical Zn status in animals; however, there may be species differences in whether plasma Zn or erythrocyte Zn is the most reliable.[4] Erythrocyte Zn is potentially less impacted by stressors but also less sensitive to depletion than serum/plasma Zn.[4,46,47]

Low serum Zn can reflect dietary deficiency, but deficiency can still be present when serum Zn levels seem adequate.[1] Isolated low serum Zn values may also represent stress.[4] However, this may be further investigated if plasma is used, because plasma Cu rises with stress, so a ratio with low plasma Zn but high plasma Cu would be more likely due to stress, whereas low plasma Zn with normal plasma Cu is more likely caused by a dietary Zn deficiency. This ratio, however, does not work with serum mineral analysis as serum Cu is inaccurate.[4]

If analyzing Zn using serum, the serum should be separated from the clot within 4 to 6 hours to reduce the chance of a falsely elevated serum Zn, caused by leaching from red blood cells.[1] Trace mineral-specific blood tubes should be used whenever possible to reduce Zn contamination from tube tops (eg, red tops), which use lubricants containing Zn.[48] If you want to test for Zn with serum, collect in trace mineral-specific tubes spun within 4 to 6 hours of collection. Alternatively, if possible, but especially if also analyzing Cu, measure plasma Zn using a blue trace mineral tube with added ethylenediaminetetraacetic acid (EDTA) for obtaining plasma.

COPPER

Copper (Cu) functions as an essential structural micromineral in macromolecules and several enzymes.[1] Cu also influences reproductive health, bone development, cellular respiration, iron metabolism, and connective tissue development, pigmentation and has antioxidative properties.[4] Sources of high natural dietary Cu include shellfish, organ meats, nuts, and some fertilized plants, but most cereal grains and forages are low in Cu.[49]

Cu deficiency tends to be more prevalent in animals than toxicity, with ruminants being more susceptible to Cu-responsive disorders than nonruminants.[45] If a deficiency is suspected based on clinical presentation, supplementation for Cu-deficient animals can help reverse some of the negative effects of low Cu, especially with hematological manifestations (ie, anemia).[50]

Cu toxicosis can either be acute or chronic depending on the species, supplementation, and relative concentrations of other dietary trace minerals (ie, S, Mo, Zn, and Ca), which impact Cu absorption.[51] Plasma Cu can also be falsely elevated from stressors such as infectious disease or vaccinations because the Cu-containing protein ceruloplasmin acts as an acute phase protein.[52] Ceruloplasmin and Cu levels are highly correlated[53,54]; however, ceruloplasmin levels have been shown to increase with high dietary starch intake.[55] Ceruloplasmin can be measured in addition to plasma Cu but should likely not replace it. Cu status can be lowered by high dietary iron, Mn, and Mo when sulfur is present.[4]

The Cu status of an animal would ideally be evaluated through plasma and not serum. Cu is largely found in ceruloplasmin in circulation.[56] When serum samples are taken ceruloplasmin and Cu-containing proteins become integrated in the clot, causing misleadingly lower serum Cu concentrations than that of plasma.[1] The amount of Cu incorporated into the serum clot varies between individuals and species. Plasma is the more reliable indicator of Cu status.[57] Therefore, a blue trace mineral tube with added EDTA for obtaining plasma would be the best choice.

MANGANESE

The micromineral manganese (Mn) is a component of enzymatic reactions, bone development and maintenance, and fertility.[1,4] Mn is also noted for being involved in intermediary metabolism, antioxidation, immune function, cell regulation, connective tissue development, and blood clotting.[4]

Owing to Mn being distributed throughout the body in low concentrations and the lack of apparent strong homeostatic controls, most animals will only manifest Mn deficiency or toxicity for short periods of time, if either is encountered under normal environmental circumstances.[58] While rare, Mn deficiency and toxicity can still occur.

Mn deficiency tends to occur due to a lack of bioavailable dietary Mn, mineral antagonisms, or high amounts of inhibitory phytate and fiber in the animal's diet. Avian species tend to be more susceptible to manganese deficiency through inadequate dietary sources such as seeds.[45] Dietary Mn supplementation can reverse Mn deficiency and prevent reoccurrence.[4] High levels of Mn in the diet can also inhibit the gastrointestinal absorption of iron and Zn due to shared intestinal transporters.[59,60]

Although high levels of Mn can be associated with liver malfunction and central nervous system disorders,[58,61] they are more commonly an artifact of hemolysis in the blood sample. Therefore, high Mn values, without context of other assays cannot be trusted. Primarily carried in red blood cells, Mn in circulation is generally low.[1] In a non-hemolyzed sample, serum Mn is more reliable for evaluating Mn status than whole blood Mn, which is nonresponsive to diet, therefore, not helpful.[1] Samples collected for serum Mn should be separated from the clot within 2 to 3 hours after collection to reduce the chances of Mn leaching from red blood cells.[1] A trace mineral blue tube is best for serum analysis of Mn.

MOLYBDENUM

Molybdenum (Mo), a micromineral, is most noted for its effects on Cu metabolism in ruminants[62] and activating xanthine oxidoreductase, aldehyde oxidase, and sulfite oxidase. It is also known for activating enzymes critical for regulating superoxide radicals that cause muscle damage and impair iron metabolism.[1,4,63] Dietary Mo can be found in pasture plants, but is low in cereal grains, and unlikely to be deficient.[4] Supplementation needs are unlikely.

Dietary Mo is soluble and readily absorbed, so Mo status can be reliably assessed with serum measurement.[64] Mo serum values are generally evaluated when there is a potential for toxicosis or secondary Cu deficiency.[65] High serum Mo is concerning as this can reflect the presence of oxythiomolybdates.[1] These chelated complexes bind Cu making it unavailable, masking Cu deficiency despite elevated serum Cu.[66]

COBALT AND VITAMIN B$_{12}$

Cobalt (Co) is a structural necessity for vitamin B$_{12}$, an integral part of the folate cycle, red blood cell formation, and fatty acid metabolism. Hindgut fermenting exotic small mammals, such as guinea pigs and rabbits, rely on cecotrophy, or the consumption of cecotropes, to obtain their daily vitamin B$_{12}$ requirements.[67] In all animals, stomach acid is needed for processing Co and vitamin B$_{12}$ before absorption. Co and B$_{12}$ can therefore be a concern in older animals where a lack of stomach acid is available for nutrient processing and absorption.

Vitamin B$_{12}$ toxicity has not been reported but Co toxicity could be a concern if dietary supplementation is excessive.[1] Co and B$_{12}$ deficiencies are more common than toxicity. Low serum vitamin B$_{12}$ indicates deficiency; however, normal or even high serum values do not rule out deficiency.[68] Serum Co is unfortunately not an ideal indicator of Co status in most circumstances. Instead, measuring serum transcobalamin (a form of B$_{12}$) can better reflect body Co status and the successful supplementation of either B$_{12}$ or Co.[4] A better, but more invasive, measure of Co and B$_{12}$ would require analysis of a liver biopsy, where low B$_{12}$ reflects suboptimal Co intake.[4] If a Co deficiency is present, a decline in serum vitamin B$_{12}$ should also be expected.[69] Co deficiency can be reversed through appropriate supplementation, as serum Co will increase with direct supplementation of the mineral[70]; however, it may be more efficient to consider B$_{12}$ supplementation to support both B$_{12}$ and Co needs.

SELENIUM

Selenium (Se) functions are widespread, mainly related to cellular defense. Se serves in antioxidant defense from lipid peroxidation, working in conjunction with vitamin E in detoxification and protection. Se directly impacts cell-mediated immunity including neutrophil proliferation and subsequent reactive oxygen species defense and allows thyroid hormone activation.[71] Se deficiency can lead to white muscle disease, reproductive problems, immunologic compromise, thyroid, and kidney dysfunction.[4] Se is also linked to the status of vitamin E in the body, reflecting the fight against oxidant challenges and stressors. During times of oxidant crises, healthy Se levels will keep vitamin E from being exhausted and decreasing.

Serum Se and whole blood Se can be used as markers of circulating body Se. Serum indicates short-term circulation, whereas whole blood indicates long-term storage, though the functional indicator of Se in the body would be measurement of glutathione peroxidase.[4]

Dietary Se levels directly impact circulating Se, as demonstrated in a variety of species.[72–74] Low levels of Se in circulation can indicate both use in the body and potential low dietary Se content. However, high levels of Se in the serum would prompt a dietary investigation. Se-rich foods are primarily from animal sources, as Se is abundant in muscle tissue, and Se values increase with higher trophic levels. Plant Se depends on soil Se content across the world, leading to extreme variation. Therefore, hay and other plants grown in different parts of the country have greatly varying Se levels.

For example, wild pikas were found to be Se deficient due to low Se plants in the Rocky Mountains.[75]

The form of dietary Se affects absorption and utilization.[4] Se can be offered as sodium selenite or as organic forms bound to methionine and carried in yeast. Toxicoses can occur from careless feeding of supplements or high-Se food items. Therefore, Se is tightly regulated in complete pelleted feeds by the US Food and Drug Administration, and most pelleted feeds are formulated to meet the minimum requirement for Se across species.[72]

IODINE

Iodine (I) functions as a constituent of thyroid hormones, with the majority of I residing in the thyroid gland. I content varies greatly across foodstuffs,[4] creating a possible need for supplementation. When clinical symptoms lead to suspicions of I dysregulation, serum I values can be misleading. Inorganic I reflects dietary intake in the short term and is rapidly excreted from the kidneys. Protein-bound iodine (PBI) is a better indicator of body I status in line with thyroid hormone T4.[1] Total serum I (PBI + inorganic I), can overestimate I status if diets have cyanogenic goitrogens present. A high ratio of serum I to T4 indicates exposure to dietary goitrogens.[4] I deficiency disorders are more common than toxicity, as many foods have the potential for goitrogen content , for example, unheated soybeans, white clover, and *Brassica* species such as kale.[4] I dietary supplementation can treat I deficiencies but be wary targeting normal ranges for your species in question. Toxicity is rare unless feeds with seaweed, or algae derivatives are a large proportion of the diet.[76] Se deficiency can also induce I deficiency.[77]

VITAMIN A

Vitamin A functions metabolically in critical ways to support vision, cellular differentiation, gene expression, growth, innate and adaptive immunity, bone development, and reproduction.[3] Vitamin A is the generic descriptor for compounds exhibiting the biological activity of retinol (ie, retinoids) and some provitamin A carotenoids.[3] It is often found bound to fatty acid esters such as palmitate in animal products, but can also be bound to proteins, especially when in the carotenoid form found in plants. Vitamin A is fat-soluble, meaning that the presence of fat is needed for absorption. Carotenoids such as beta-carotene are cleaved into vitamin A for absorption by an enzyme that may not be present in the gut of all species. Notable taxa that lack this enzyme include cat species and potentially amphibians.[8,78] When a vitamin A deficiency is suspected in an exotic species, it is wise to examine the diet for form and source of vitamin A and consider the fat content of the diet, as there may be challenges to absorption. For amphibian species, vitamin A deficiency can manifest as short tongue syndrome; topical, rather than oral, vitamin A supplementation at low doses can be an effective treatment, but dose must be carefully calculated and frequency of administration carefully considered avoiding toxicity.[79,80] Birds also commonly suffer from vitamin A deficiency if fed a high-fat seed-only or majority seed-based diet.[81]

Hyper- and hypovitaminosis A are common across species, but especially in birds, reptiles, and amphibians. Serum/plasma vitamin A will allow diagnosis of hypervitaminosis A but may not be a true indicator of low status unless severely deficient because of the tissue storage capacity for vitamin A. Diet supplementation of vitamin A based on serum values alone should be administered with caution, and administration dose should be conservative, as high levels may quickly swing an animal toward toxicity.

VITAMIN D$_3$

Vitamin D is unique in that it can come from dietary sources and also be created in the skin of most animals in a chemical reaction involving ultraviolet (UV) radiation from the sun. Human research has questioned the universality of sun exposure satisfying requirements dependent on seasonality, location in the world, and even time of day of exposure.[82] As vitamin D is critical for growth and interdependent with Ca and P, growing animals are especially sensitive to deficiency. Cholecalciferol (D$_3$) is a fat-soluble vitamin with the potential for toxicity on overdose in the diet. Before considering vitamin D supplementation, consider the form of vitamin D already in the diet, sun, or UV exposure in the animal and even the fat content of the diet. Dietary supplementation may be needed even in the presence of seemingly adequate lighting, as UV lamps can degrade in intensity with time.[83]

Vitamin D also serves functions such as vitamin A in regulating gene expression through nuclear receptors impacting transcription and functions as a hormone to bind to membrane receptors on target tissues and activates a signal transduction pathway. Basically, these vitamins have far-reaching impacts when they are dysregulated. Metabolic bone disease due to vitamin D deficiency has been documented in multiple species.[84] There have also been many documented cases of toxicity.[22,85]

The major circulating form of vitamin D, important for function, is 25-OH vitamin D$_3$ — this is what should be measured in serum. Owing to differences in analytical methods and standardization, reported vitamin D values across laboratories vary, and reference ranges across species may warrant a critical eye. We recommend using established commercial laboratories with strong quality assurance/quality control (QA/QC), who ideally specialize in vitamin analyses, including vitamin D. Other forms of vitamin D are 25-OH vitamin D$_2$, 1,25(OH)$_2$ vitamin D (the active form), and 24,25(OH)$_2$ vitamin D2/D3 forms (catabolism products). These forms are very different in function and amount in circulation and are generally separate costly analyses. If you are concerned about vitamin D toxicity or deficiency, make sure you request the correct analysis, at a trusted facility.

VITAMIN C

It is unlikely that there will be a need to assess vitamin C status in most species, the exception being the guinea pig due to its inability to synthesize ascorbic acid from glucose.[86,87] If a vitamin C deficiency is suspected due to symptoms or evaluation of diet, serum or plasma levels may help to confirm a diagnosis. Ganguly and colleagues[88] reported serum levels of 0.21 mg/dL in guinea pigs fed a deficient diet for 3 weeks and values of 0.007 mg/dL in those fed a deficient diet for 4 weeks.

Dietary levels of vitamin C in the guinea pig may also affect the serum levels of other nutrients. Vitamin C deficiency can increase serum Cu,[89] whereas high doses of vitamin C can decrease serum Cu levels.[90] Serum Fe levels may also be directly influenced by dietary vitamin C levels.[89] Recommended dietary levels of vitamin C for guinea pigs are 20 to 30 mg/kg diet.[91] Dietary levels in excess of 25 mg/100 g body weight were found to interfere with Cu status.[89]

VITAMIN E

Vitamin E (α-tocopherol) is known for its primary role in antioxidative defense systems of the body but also impacts gene expression and enzyme regulation.[3] Vitamin E deficiency is more common than toxicity, with toxicity far rarer than its fat-soluble counterpart's vitamin A and D. Most species tolerate high levels of vitamin E in the diet with no ill effect. Vitamin E can be found in fats, oils, nuts, seeds, certain fresh pastures,

Table 1
Brief reference tool[a] for interpretation of serum mineral analytes

Mineral	Is Serum… The Best Measure of Total Body Status?	…Meaningful Relating Most to Which Nutrients?	Sample Preferred for Analysis	Wide Range of Potential Normality	Direct Reflection of Dietary Intake	Commonly Above or Below Reference Range?	Common Association: Deficiency or Toxicity?	Body Reserve Present
Ca	Yes	Yes: Vit D, P, Mg, Fe	Serum; ionized Ca for birds/reptiles/critically ill	No	No: except immediately after Ca intake	Both	Both	Yes: Bone
P	Yes	Yes: Vit D, Ca, Fe, Zn, Cu, Mo	Serum	Yes	Yes: caveat phytate	Above	Both	No
Mg	No	Yes: K, Ca	Serum	No	Yes	Below	Deficiency	Yes
Zn	Yes	Yes: Cu, P, Fe	Serum or plasma	No	Yes: caveat can mask body deficiency	Below	Deficiency	Yes: Skeletal muscle
Fe	No	Yes: Vit B$_{12}$, Cu, P, Vit C hematology	Liver; transferrin saturation; ferritin	Yes	No: multifactorial	Both	Deficiency; except for species prone to iron overload	Yes: red blood cells (RBC)/liver
Cu	No	Yes: Zn, Se, Fe, Mo, S	Plasma; serum misleading	Yes	Yes	Below	Deficiency	Yes
Mn	Yes	Yes: Fe, Zn	Whole blood or serum	No	No	Above: likely hemolysis artifact	Neither	No
Se	No	Yes: Vit E	Serum	Yes	Yes	Both	Deficiency	No
Mo	Yes	Yes: Cu	Serum	No	Yes	Above	Toxicity	No
Co	No	Yes: B$_{12}$, hematology	Serum transcobalamin	No	Yes	Below	Deficiency	Yes
I	No	Y: Se, Co	Serum	Yes	No	Below	Deficiency	Yes

[a] These are generalized highlight responses and may not cover all aspects and exceptions for these micronutrients. Please see the Sullivan et al. 2023 chapter and other more in-depth references for details and explanations.

Table 2
Brief reference tool[a] for interpretation of serum vitamin analytes

Vitamin	Is Serum.... ...The Best Measure of Total Body Status?	...Meaningful Relating Most to Which Nutrients?	Ideal Form for Analysis	Wide Range of Potential Normality	Direct Reflection of Dietary Intake	Commonly Above or Below Reference Range?	Common Association: Deficiency or Toxicity?	Body Reserve Present
A	Yes	Yes: Vit D, Fe, I	Retinol	Yes	Yes	Both	Both	Yes: liver/adipose
D	Yes	Yes: Ca, P, Mg,	$25(OH)D_3$	Yes	Yes: also, from skin/sun	Both	Both, deficiency more common	Yes: liver/adipose
E	Yes	Yes: Se, Fe, Cu, Zn	α-tocopherol	Yes	Yes	Below	Deficiency	Yes: liver/adipose
C	Yes	Yes: Fe, Cu	Ascorbic acid	No	Yes	Neither	Deficiency	No

[a] These are generalized highlight responses and may not cover all aspects and exceptions for these micronutrients. Please see the Sullivan et al. 2023 chapter and other more in-depth references for details and explanations.

complete feeds, and green leafy vegetables.[92] Supplemental α-tocopherol is the only form of vitamin E that can be used to reverse the effects of vitamin E deficiency.[93]

Vitamin E deficiency in plasma and serum can directly reflect lack of dietary vitamin E, a Se deficiency, lipid malabsorption, or a diet high in polyunsaturated fatty acids.[3] Some laboratories struggle to measure very low values of vitamin E, so communication is warranted if the results come back "not detected" to ensure this meant it was below the limit of detection rather than a laboratory error.

Circulating serum vitamin E in serum and/or plasma can fluctuate with dietary intake, fat reserves, and body use which are poorly understood across exotic species.[94] Over 90% of vitamin E is stored in fat reserves with excess regulated via excretion through the feces. Other non-α forms of dietary vitamin E do not serve the same function (β, γ, or δ tocopherol, or tocotrienols).

SUMMARY

When interpreting nutrient analytical reports, it is important to always look at the bigger picture and not get too caught up in overinterpreting serum micronutrients as above or below a particular species' reference range (**Tables 1** and **2**). When deciding whether to analyze for these micronutrients, know what you are testing for and why, the factors that may affect your results (eg, diet, other minerals, disease states), and how you will interpret results received. Further, be sure to have a good understanding of sample handling, processing, and laboratory analytical methods so that you can better trust analytical results. Dietary supplementation can be helpful in some cases, but it is more important to evaluate the current diet and holistically assess what may be interfering with healthy micronutrient absorption or metabolism.

CLINICS CARE POINTS

- Serum micronutrients, such as fat-soluble vitamins, calcium, and iron, can be forgiving of an inconsistent diet due to nutrient storage within the body.

- For birds and reptiles in active reproduction and any animal in a disease state, ionized calcium will give a more accurate assessment of status than total serum calcium.

- Dietary intake of calcium does not have a large impact on serum calcium in mammals except directly after meals including calcium. Phytate is a form of phosphorus that binds other minerals including calcium, iron, and zinc, affecting their absorption and digestion.

- Plasma copper is preferred over serum copper for assessment and is elevated when animals are under stress.

- Serum iron does not necessarily reflect dietary iron in all species, nor does it always reflect when iron is elevated in the body. Measuring ferritin and transferrin saturation in serum can aid toxicity assessment when possible. Low serum iron may have many causes; therefore, iron supplementation should be considered cautiously across species.

- Elevated serum manganese is most commonly an artifact of hemolysis, rather than diet- or metabolism-related.

- Selenium in dietary plant sources can vary widely based on where they are grown, and the diet sources should be evaluated if serum selenium is either very low or very high.

- Vitamin E deficiency with low serum vitamin E is more common than toxicity.

- Vitamin A deficiency and toxicity can manifest across species differently but is clearly reflected in serum retinol. Dietary form of vitamin A or provitamin carotenoids can influence absorption across species.

ACKNOWLEDGMENTS

The authors would like to thank Dr Heidi Bissell for her editing expertise and support.

DISCLOSURE

The authors declare that they have no relevant or material financial interests that relate to the research described in this paper.

REFERENCES

1. Herdt TH, Hoff B. The use of blood analysis to evaluate trace mineral status in ruminant livestock. Vet Clin N Am: Food Anim Pract. 2011;27(2):255–83.
2. McDowell LR. Vitamins in animal and human nutrition. Ames: Iowa State University Press; 2000.
3. Combs GF Jr, McClung JP. The vitamins: fundamental aspects in nutrition and health. Cambridge: Academic press; 2017.
4. Suttle NF. Mineral nutrition of livestock. 5th edition. Cambridge: Cabi; 2022.
5. Hokamp JA, Nabity MB. Renal biomarkers in domestic species. Vet Clin Pathol 2016;45(1):28–56.
6. Chan LN, Mike LA. The science and practice of micronutrient supplementations in nutritional anemia: An evidence-based review. J Parenter Enteral Nutr 2014; 38(6):656–72.
7. Golden MH. Specific deficiencies versus growth failure: type I and type II nutrients. J Nutr Environ Med 1996;6(3):301–8.
8. Morris JG. Idiosyncratic nutrient requirements of cats appear to be diet-induced evolutionary adaptations. Nutr Res Rev 2002;15(1):153–68.
9. Allen ME, Oftedal OT, Baer DJ. The feeding and nutrition of carnivores. In: Kleinman DG, Allen ME, Thompson KV, et al, editors. Wild mammals in captivity. Chicago: University of Chicago Press; 1996. p. 139–47.
10. de Matos R. Calcium metabolism in birds. Vet Clin North Am Exot Anim Pract 2008;11(1):59–82.
11. Forman DT, Lorenzo L. Ionized calcium: its significance and clinical usefulness. Ann Clin Lab Sci 1991;21:297–304.
12. Dennis PM, Bennett RA, Harr KE, et al. Plasma concentrations of ionized calcium in healthy iguanas. J Am Vet Med Assoc 2001;219:326–8.
13. Hoopes LA. Elasmobranch mineral and vitamin requirements. The Elasmobranch Husbandry Manual II 2017;135.
14. Goldstein DA. Serum Calcium. Clinical methods: the history, physical and laboratory examinations 3rd ed. 1990.
15. Houillier P, Froissart M, Maruani G, et al. What serum calcium can tell us and what it can't. Nephrol Dial Transplant 2006;21(1):29–32.
16. Dessauer HC. Blood chemistry of reptiles: physiological and evolutionary aspects. Biology of the Reptile 1970;3(1):1–72.
17. Torres DA, Freitas MB, Gonçalves RV. Changes in bone turnover and calcium homeostasis during pregnancy and lactation in mammals: a meta-analysis. Reprod Fertil Dev 2018;30(5):681–8.
18. Siegel A, Walton RM. Hematology and biochemistry of small mammals. Ferrets, Rabbits and Rodents 2020;569.
19. Eckermann-Ross C. Hormonal regulation and calcium metabolism in the rabbit. Vet Clin North Am Exot Anim Pract 2008;11:139–52.
20. Blas CD, Wiseman J, editors. Nutrition of the rabbit. 2nd edition. India: Cabi; 2010.

21. Carmel B, Johnson R. Nutritional and metabolic diseases. In: Donely B, Monks D, Johnson R, et al, editors. Reptile medicine and surgery in clinical practice. Oxford: Wiley Blackwell; 2018.
22. DeClementi C, Sobczak BR. Common rodenticide toxicoses in small animals. Vet Clin North Am Small Anim Pract 2012;42(2):349–60.
23. LaDouceur EEB, Murphy BG, Garner MM, et al. Osteomalacia With Hyperostosis in Captive Lesser Hedgehog Tenrecs (*Echinops telfairi*). Vet Path 2020;57(6): 885–8.
24. Schenck PA, Chew DJ. Calcium: Total or ionized? Vet Clin North Am Small Anim Pract 2008;38(3):497–502.
25. Schenck PA, Chew DJ. Prediction of serum ionized calcium concentration by serum total calcium measurement in cats. Can J Vet Res 2010;74(3):209–13.
26. Byrnes MC, Huyhn K, Helmer SD, et al. A comparison of corrected serum calcium levels to ionized calcium levels among critically ill surgical patients. Am J Surg 2005;189(3):310–4.
27. Fowler A, Hansen T, Strasinger L, et al. Phosphorus digestibility and phytate degradation by yearlings and mature horses. J Anim Sci 2015;93:5735–42.
28. Humer E, Zebeli Q. Phytate in feed ingredients and potentials for improving the utilization of phosphorus in ruminant nutrition. Anim Feed Sci Technol 2015; 209:1–15.
29. Fawcett WJ, Haxby EJ, Male DA. Magnesium: Physiology and pharmacology. Br J Anaesth 1999;83:302–20.
30. Reinhart RA. Magnesium metabolism: A review with special reference to the relationship between intracellular content and serum levels. Arch Intern Med 1988; 148:2415–20.
31. Ahmed F, Mohammed A. Magnesium: the forgotten electrolyte—a review on hypomagnesemia. Med Sci 2019;7(4):56.
32. Martens H, Schweigel M. Pathophysiology of grass tetany and other hypomagnesemias: implications for clinical management. Vet Clin N Am: Food Anim Pract. 2000;16(2):339–68.
33. Knutson M, Wessling-Resnick M. Iron metabolism in the reticuloendothelial system. Crit Rev Biochem Mol Biol 2003;38:61–88.
34. Klopfleisch R, Olias P. The pathology of comparative animal models of human haemochromatosis. J Comp Pathol 2012;10:1–20.
35. Cacoub P, Vandewalle C, Peoc'h K. Using transferrin saturation as a diagnostic criterion for iron deficiency: A systematic review. Crit Rev Clin Lab Sci 2019; 56(8):526–32.
36. Elsayed ME, Sharif MU, Stack AG. Transferrin saturation: a body iron biomarker. Adv Clin Chem 2016;75:71–97.
37. Sullivan KE, Mylniczenko ND, Nelson SE Jr, et al. Practical management of iron overload disorder in black rhinoceros (Diceros bicornis). Animals 2020;10(11): 1991.
38. Smith JE, Chavey S, Miller RE. Iron metabolism in captive black (Diceros bicornis) and white (Ceratotherium simum) rhinoceroses. J Zoo Wildl Med 1995;26:525–31.
39. Timoshnikov VA, Kobzeva TV, Polyakov NE, et al. Redox interactions of vitamin C and iron: Inhibition of the pro-oxidant activity by Deferiprone. Int J Mol Sci 2020 May 31;21(11):3967.
40. Theil EC. Iron, ferritin, and nutrition. Annu Rev Nutr 2004;24:327–43.
41. Zielińska-Dawidziak M. Plant ferritin—a source of iron to prevent its deficiency. Nutrients 2015;7(2):1184–201.

42. King JC, Cousins RJ. Zinc. In: Ross AC, Caballero B, Cousins RJ, et al, editors. Modern nutrition in health and disease. 11th edition. Burlington: Jones & Bartlett Learning; 2014. p. 189–205.

43. Ross AC, Caballero B, Cousins RJ, et al, editors. Modern nutrition in health and disease. Jones & Bartlett Learning; 2020.

44. Hambidge KM, Miller LV, Westcott JE, et al. Zinc bioavailability and homeostasis. Am J Clin Nutr 2010;91(5):1478S–83S.

45. Underwood EJ, Suttle NF. The mineral nutrition of livestock. 3rd edition. Cambridge: Cabi; 2004.

46. Choi S, Lui X, Pan Z. Zinc deficiency and cellular oxidative stress: prognostic implications in cardiovascular diseases. Acta Pharm Sin 2018;39:1120–32.

47. Lukaski HC. Low dietary zinc decreases erythrocyte carbonic anhydrase activities and impairs cardiorespiratory function in men during exercise. Am J Clin Nutr 2005;81(5):1045–51.

48. Keyzer JJ, Oosting E, Wolthers BG, et al. Zinc in plasma and serum: influence of contamination due to the collection tubes. Pharm Weekbl 1983;5:248–51.

49. Cromwell GL. Copper as a nutrient for animals. In: Richardson HW. Handbook of copper compounds and applications. New York: Marcel Dekker, Inc; 1997. p. 177–202.

50. Myint ZW, Oo TH, Thein KZ, et al. Copper deficiency anemia. Ann Hematol 2018; 97:1527–34.

51. Kimberling CV. Jensen and Swift's diseases of Sheep. 3rd Edition. Philadelphia: Lea & Febiger; 1988.

52. Suttle NF. Meeting the copper requirements of ruminants. In: Garnsworthy PC, Cole DJA, editors. Recent advances in animal nutrition. Nottingham: Nottingham University Press; 1994. p. 173–88.

53. Legleiter LR, Spears JW. Plasma diamine oxidase: a biomarker of copper deficiency in the bovine. J An Sci 2007;85:2198–204.

54. Laven RA, Lawrence KE. Analysis of the value of measurement of the activity of caeruloplasmin as an alternative to measurement of the concentration of elemental copper in plasma and serum of farmed red deer. N Z Vet J 2010;58: 334–8.

55. McCaughern JH, Mackenzie AM, Sinclair LA. Dietary starch concentration alters reticular pH, hepatic copper concentration, and performance in lactating Holstein-Friesian dairy cows receiving added dietary sulfur and molybdenum. J Dairy Sci 2020;103:9024–36.

56. Prohaska JR. Copper. In: Prohaska JR, Bowman BA, Russell RM, editors. Present knowledge in nutrition. Washington DC: International Life Sciences Institute; 2006. p. 458–70.

57. Laven RA, Smith SL. Copper deficiency in sheep: an assessment of relationship between concentrations of copper in serum and plasma. N Z Vet J 2008;56(6): 334–8.

58. Keen CL, Ensunsa JL, Clegg MS. Manganese metabolism in animals and humans including the toxicity of manganese. Met Ions Biol Syst 2000;37(2):89–121.

59. Hansen SL, Spears JW. Impact of copper deficiency in cattle on proteins involved in iron metabolism. FASEB J 2008;22:443–5.

60. Lui Q, Barker S, Knutson MD. Iron and manganese transport in mammalian systems. Biochim Biophys Acta Mol Cell Res 2021;1868(1):118890.

61. Hauser RA, Zesiewicz TA, Rosemurgy AS, et al. Manganese intoxication and chronic liver failure. Ann Neurol 1994;36(6):871–5.

62. Underwood EJ. Trace elements in human and animal nutrition. New York: Academic Press; 1977.

63. Johnson JL. Molybdenum. In: O'Dell BL, Sunde RA, editors. Handbook of nutritionally essential mineral elements. New York: Marcel Dekker; 1997. p. 413–38.

64. Kincaid RL. Assessment of trace mineral status of ruminants: A review. J Anim Sci 2000;77(E):1–10.

65. Turnlund JR, Keyes WR. Plasma molybdenum reflects dietary molybdenum intake. J Nutr Biochem 2004;15(2):90–5.

66. Suttle NF. The interactions between copper, molybdenum, and sulphur in ruminant nutrition. Annu Rev Nutr 1991;11:121–40.

67. Quesenberry KE, Carpenter JW. Ferrets, rabbits, and rodents: clinical medicine and surgery: includes sugar gliders and hedgehogs. 2nd ed. St. Louis: Saunders; 2004.

68. Andres E, Serraj K, Zhu J, et al. The pathophysiology of elevated vitamin B12 in clinical practice. QJM 2013;106(6):505–15.

69. Stangl GI, Schwarz FK, Jahn B, et al. Cobalt–deficiency–induced hyperhomocysteinaemia and oxidative status of cattle. Br J Nutr 2000;83(1):3–6.

70. Vellema P, Moll L, Barkema HW, et al. Effect of cobalt supplementation on serum vitamin B12 levels, weight gain and survival rate in lambs grazing cobalt-deficient pastures. Vet Q 1997;19(1):1–5.

71. Hoffmann PR, Berry MJ. The influence of selenium on immune responses. Mol Nutr Food Res 2008;52(11):1273–80.

72. Ullrey DE. Basis for regulation of selenium supplements in animal diets. J Anim Sci 1992;70(12):3922–7.

73. Montgomery JB, Wichtel JJ, Wichtel MG, et al. The efficacy of selenium treatment of forage for the correction of selenium deficiency in horses. Anim Feed Sci Technol 2011;170(1–2):63–71.

74. Sikarskie JG, Van Veen TS, Ullrey DE, et al. Comparative serum selenium values for ranched and free-ranging American bison (Bison bison). J Zoo Wildl Med 1989;34–8.

75. Palmer KM, Stanton NL, Ben-David M, et al. Are pikas exposed to and affected by selenium deficiency? J Wildl Dis 2007;43(3):475–84.

76. Rey-Crespo F, López-Alonso M, Miranda M. The use of seaweed from the Galician coast as a mineral supplement in organic dairy cattle. Animal 2014;8(4): 580–6.

77. Mitchell JH, Nicol F, Beckett GJ. Selenium and iodine deficiencies: effects on brain and brown adipose tissue selenoenzyme activity and expression. J Endocrinol 1997;155(2):255–63.

78. Clugston RD, Blaner WS. Vitamin A (retinoid) metabolism and action: What we know and what we need to know about amphibians. Zoo Biol 2014;33(6):527–35.

79. Sim RR, Sullivan KE, Valdes EV, et al. A comparison of oral and topical vitamin A supplementation in African foam-nesting frogs (Chiromantis xerampelina). J Zoo Wildl Med 2010;41(3):456–60.

80. Rodriguez CE, Pessier AP. Pathologic changes associated with suspected hypovitaminosis A in amphibians under managed care. Zoo Biol 2014;33(6):508–15.

81. Hess L, Mauldin G, Rosenthal K. Estimated nutrient content of diets commonly fed to pet birds. Vet Rec 2002;150(13):399–404.

82. Wacker M, Holick MF. Sunlight and vitamin D: A global perspective for health. Derm Endocrinol 2013;5(1):51–108.

83. Wood MN, Soltis J, Sullivan KE, et al. UV irradiance effects on Komodo dragon (Varanus komodoensis) vitamin D3, egg production, and behavior: A case study. Zoo Biol 2023;1–10.

84. Uhl EW. The pathology of vitamin D deficiency in domesticated animals: An evolutionary and comparative overview. Int J Paleopathol 2018;23:100–9.

85. Wimsatt J, Marks SL, Campbell TW, et al. Dietary vitamin D toxicity in a household of pot-bellied pigs (Sus scrofa). J Vet Intern Med 1998;12(1):42–4.

86. Harkness JE, Murray KA, Wagner JE. Biology and Diseases of Guinea Pigs. Laboratory Animal Medicine 2002;203.

87. Quesenberry KE. Guinea pigs. Vet Clin N Am: Small Anim Pract. 1994;24(1): 67–87.

88. Ganguly R, Durieux MF, Waldman RH. Macrophage function in vitamin C deficient guinea pigs. Am J Clin Nutr 1976;29(7):762–5.

89. Milne DB, Omaye ST. Effect of Vitamin C on copper and iron metabolism in the Guinea Pig. Int J Vitam Nutr Res 1980;50(3):301–8.

90. Kadrabová J, Madaric A, Ginter E. Zinc and copper in the tissues and serum of cadmium intoxicated guinea-pigs: influence of vitamin C. Physiol Res 1993;42(4): 261–6.

91. Garner-Richardson V. Guinea pig nutrition. Vet Nurse 2012;3(5):274–82.

92. Traber MG. Micronutrient Information Center Vitamin E. Linus Pauling Institute Oregon State University. 2015. Available at: https://lpi.oregonstate.edu/mic/vitamins/vitamin-E. Accessed May 1, 2023.

93. Traber MG. Vitamin E inadequacy in humans: causes and consequences. Adv Nutr 2014;5(5):503–14.

94. Dierenfeld ES, Traber MG. Vitamin E status of exotic animals compared with livestock and domestics. In: Packer L, Fuchs J, editors. Vitamin E in health and disease. New York: Marcel Dekker Inc; 1993. p. 345–70.

Moving?

Make sure your subscription moves with you!

To notify us of your new address, find your **Clinics Account Number** (located on your mailing label above your name), and contact customer service at:

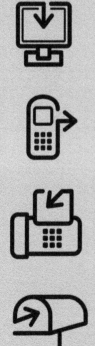

Email: **journalscustomerservice-usa@elsevier.com**

800-654-2452 (subscribers in the U.S. & Canada)
314-447-8871 (subscribers outside of the U.S. & Canada)

Fax number: 314-447-8029

Elsevier Health Sciences Division
Subscription Customer Service
3251 Riverport Lane
Maryland Heights, MO 63043

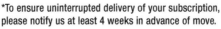

Printed and bound by CPI Group (UK) Ltd, Croydon, CR0 4YY

03/10/2024

01040470-0012